Rosangelis Del Lama Soares

Living with Phenylketonuria

Rosangelis Del Lama Soares

Living with Phenylketonuria

Maternal perception and that of the multi-professional team

ScienciaScripts

Imprint

Any brand names and product names mentioned in this book are subject to trademark, brand or patent protection and are trademarks or registered trademarks of their respective holders. The use of brand names, product names, common names, trade names, product descriptions etc. even without a particular marking in this work is in no way to be construed to mean that such names may be regarded as unrestricted in respect of trademark and brand protection legislation and could thus be used by anyone.

Cover image: www.ingimage.com

This book is a translation from the original published under ISBN 978-613-9-66630-0.

Publisher:
Sciencia Scripts
is a trademark of
Dodo Books Indian Ocean Ltd. and OmniScriptum S.R.L publishing group

120 High Road, East Finchley, London, N2 9ED, United Kingdom
Str. Armeneasca 28/1, office 1, Chisinau MD-2012, Republic of Moldova, Europe
Printed at: see last page
ISBN: 978-620-8-05264-5

PREFACE

> *"There comes a time when you have to ditch the clothes you've worn that already have the shape of your body and forget about the paths that always take you to the same places.*
> *It's time to cross over, and if we don't dare to do it, we'll have remained on the margins of ourselves forever." (Fernando Teixeira de Andrade)*

This book investigated treatment and living with Phenylketonuria (PKU) in the family through the perception of the mother and the professionals who work in the Reference Service in the state of Minas Gerais.

The research was carried out in two stages. The first investigated and discussed the repercussions of Phenylketonuria on family dynamics, from the point of view of the mothers of affected children aged between two and six. The second investigated the perception of professionals who work in the state's Reference Service on the care and treatment of the disease.

Living with phenylketonuria: the maternal perception and that of the multi-professional team, was organised into eight chapters. In the first, the Introduction contextualises the emergence of the research and points out diagnosis, treatment and living with the disease, identified in the first days of the child's life by neonatal screening.

The second chapter presents a literature review on phenylketonuria, clinical aspects of the disease, neonatal screening in the state of Minas Gerais and treatment. The third chapter highlights issues relating to the implications of the chronic disease for the family, difficulties in adhering to the diet and maintaining treatment throughout life.

The purposes of the study are described in the fourth chapter and the methodological approach in the fifth. The methodology is qualitative, using semi-structured interviews with the mothers of affected children and focus groups with the multi-professional team as data collection tools.

The results were introduced in the fifth chapter and organised and presented in chapters six and seven.

The eighth chapter deals with the Final Considerations, followed by the Bibliographical References.

ACKNOWLEDGEMENTS

To God for giving me the opportunity to carry out this work with strength, courage, patience and perseverance. A dream that I have cherished for some years, based on professional inspiration and personal maturity. A quest that has proved extraordinary and rewarding in terms of knowing, learning and sharing the unique experiences of the human being.

To the mothers interviewed for their trust, willingness to expose their lives, feelings and difficulties in living with Phenylketonuria. I would like to express my deep admiration and solidarity with these warrior mothers who go to great lengths to look after their children and live for them so that they are happy and able to fulfil their dreams.

To my husband Mário Fernando for his complicity, his affectionate and permanent presence, his unconditional love at every moment of our lives.

To my daughters Fernanda and Flávia for their solidarity, understanding and tolerance, hoping that the moments of impatience and absence become examples of commitment, responsibility and determination.

To my parents, Alcides and Sylvia, for their lessons in life, solidarity and respect for others, which were fundamental to my upbringing. Their teachings will never be forgotten.

To my brothers, Ruberval and Gilson, for their support, care and affection during the most difficult times.

To Prof Dr Marcos José Burle de Aguiar, mentor and advisor of the study, for his sensitivity, collaboration and help in making the project institutionally viable.

To Prof Dr Lúcia Maria Horta Figueiredo Goulart for agreeing to lead me down the path of qualitative methodology, always encouraging me. She was a constant, friendly, dedicated and tireless presence, masterfully guiding and monitoring all the stages of the study.

To the Centre for Action and Research in Diagnostic Support (NUPAD) of the Faculty of Medicine of the Federal University of Minas Gerais (UFMG), for the institutional and financial support and the opportunity to carry out this research, especially to the Director General, Prof. Dr José Nélio Januário.

To my dear friends and colleagues from the multi-professional team at the Phenylketonuria Outpatient Clinic, the Centre for Education and Social Support (CEAPS) and the Treatment Control Sector (SCT), whose testimonies brought this work to life. It's always a pleasure to work and share activities with a team that is integrated, dynamic, competent and committed to public health.

Finally, to phenylketonurics, with the hope that we can understand more and more about living with the disease and thus develop strategies that can help ease the difficulties of treatment and improve the quality of life of affected individuals and their families.

*"Three things remain from everything:
the certainty that we are beginning, the
certainty that we must continue and the
certainty that we can be interrupted
before we finish.*

*But you have to turn the interruption
into a new path; the fall into a
dance step; the fear into a school;
the dream into a bridge; the search
into an encounter, and then it will
have been worth existing!"*

Fernando Sabino

SUMMARY

CHAPTER 1

Introduction

"I can give you nothing that doesn't exist in you. I can't open up another world of images for you, apart from the one in your own soul. I can give you nothing but the opportunity, the impulse, the key. I'll help you make your own world visible, and that's all."

(Hermann Hesse)

Inborn errors of metabolism (IEMs) are a large group of diseases that appear mainly in the first few months of life. They are genetically determined metabolic alterations and are generally characterised by a specific deficiency in the activity of an enzyme, particularly one linked to protein synthesis (MONTEIRO; CÂNDIDO, 2006).

Phenylketonuria (PKU) is the most common IMT, with a very variable incidence in different countries and ethnic populations. In Brazil, it varies from one case per 21,000 to 13,500 live births (BRASIL, 2005).

PKU is a genetic disease of autosomal recessive inheritance, resulting from the loss or decreased activity of the liver enzyme phenylalanine hydroxylase (PHA), which catalyses the hydroxylation of phenylalanine (phe) into tyrosine (tyr). Both a deficiency of the enzyme and a defect in its cofactor tetrahydrobiopterin (BH4) lead to increased concentrations of phe in the blood and tissues. Persistent elevations of phe and its acid metabolites can cause neurological damage, the most severe form of which is irreversible mental retardation (SCRIVER; KAUFMAN, 2001).

In PKU there are no apparent abnormalities at birth, as the mother's liver protects the foetus. The blood levels of phe in phenylketonuric newborns increase in the first few weeks with protein feeding, including breast milk

(MONTEIRO; CÂNDIDO, 2006).

The neonatal screening test makes it possible to identify newborns with a suspected diagnosis of PKU and to start treatment in good time, thus preventing clinical manifestations of the disease. Carrying out the test on the third to fifth day of life allows the child to be on protein food for at least 48 hours before the blood is taken, thus reducing false-negative cases (STARLING *etal.,* 1999).

The State Newborn Screening Programme (PETN) was created in the state of Minas Gerais by resolutions 789 of 22/09/1993 and 982 of 11/03/1994, issued by the State Health Department, and has been implemented since 1993, through a partnership with the Centre for Action and Research in Diagnostic Support, a complementary body of the Faculty of Medicine of the Federal University of Minas Gerais (NUPAD-FM- UFMG). Since 2001, NUPAD has been the Reference Centre for the National Neonatal Screening Programme in Minas Gerais. It covers 100 per cent of the municipalities in Minas Gerais, covering approximately 94 per cent of live births in the state. Every month, around 22,000 screening tests are carried out, sent from around 5,000 municipal collection points, for the diagnosis of Phenylketonuria, Congenital Hypothyroidism, Sickle Cell Anaemia and Cystic Fibrosis (AGUIAR, 2004). Recently, two other diseases have been incorporated into the programme: biotinidase deficiency and congenital adrenal hyperplasia.

In addition to early diagnosis, PETN-MG is also responsible for providing specialised care, in a timely manner, for both Phenylketonuria and the other triad diseases, keeping track of the child in accordance with the protocols of the Reference Service (RS).

The incidence of PKU in Minas Gerais is one case for every 21,175 live births (MARTINS, 2005). Therefore, considering the number of blood samples processed, it is expected that every month a new patient will be identified with a suspected diagnosis and begin treatment.

The treatment is free, offered in full by the Unified Health Service (SUS) and guaranteed to all phenylketonuric patients living in Minas Gerais, whether or not they have been screened by the programme. It also includes patients with other types of hyperphenylalaninemia, such as Tetrahydrobiopterin Deficiency (BH4) and those with a late diagnosis who opt for treatment (KANUFRE *et al.*, 2001a).

In Minas Gerais, PKU treatment is centralised in Belo Horizonte, in a partnership between the State and Municipal Health Departments, NUPAD-FM-UFMG and the Hospital das Clínicas of the Federal University of Minas Gerais (HC-UFMG).

Patients are cared for by a multi-professional team made up of doctors, nutritionists, nurses, psychologists and social workers. Currently, 295 patients are being treated at the Phenylketonuria Outpatient Clinic of the Special Genetics Service of the Hospital das Clínicas (SEG-HC-UFMG), as shown in Table 1.1.

Table 1.1 **Patients being followed up at the Phenylketonuria Outpatient Clinic from 01/09/1993 to 31/10/2013, Belo Horizonte (MG)**

Diagnosis	Start of treatment		n	%
	Early n (%)	Late n (%)		
Phenylketonuria	229 (77,6)	58 (19,7)	287	97,3
BH4 deficiency		-	8	2,7
Total		-	295	100,0

Source: **NUPAD, 2013.**[1]

Of the 287 patients with Phenylketonuria, 227 (79.1%) were diagnosed with the classic form of the disease and 60 (20.9%) with Mild Phenylketonuria.

Treatment for PKU consists of a diet restricted in phe and, consequently,

---

[1] DIAGNOSTIC SUPPORT RESEARCH CENTRE - NUPAD. Database.xlsx. [personal message]. Message received by <rodls@terra.com.br>. on 12 Nov. 2013.

in natural proteins. Foods that contain proteins of high biological value, such as meat, milk and dairy products, eggs, as well as pulses, some cereals and all preparations or foods that contain them, are banned from the diet. Few

foods can be consumed freely, such as sugar, honey (after one year of age), vegetable oils and some fruits, such as acerola and lemon (KANUFRE *et aL,* 2001a).

In addition to a protein-restricted diet, treatment requires the use of a protein substitute, usually an amino acid formula, free or low in phe, in order to reach the daily recommendation of the nutrient for the affected individual. In this way, treatment allows for normal growth and neuropsychomotor development, while also helping to stabilise blood concentrations of phe (MARTINS *et aL,* 1993).

The aim of treatment is to maintain blood concentrations of phe within the limits considered safe and, at the same time, to provide adequate amounts of both phe and other macro and micronutrients (STARLING *etaL,* 1999). In most countries, including Brazil, treatment is recommended for the patient's entire life (MACDONALD, 2010; NATIONAL INSTITUTES OF HEALTH CONSENSUS, 2001).

Unlike other chronic diseases with restrictive diets, in PKU, the results of dietary transgressions and the consequent chronic increase in blood concentrations of phe are of late manifestation. Even so, these manifestations are very subjective and make it difficult to perceive the damage, which can usually only be seen at school age.

In the Phenylketonuria Outpatient Clinic at SEG-HC-UFMG, it has been noted that in the first two years of life, particularly in the first year, the children's parents and relatives manage to maintain strong adherence to treatment, motivated by fear of the diagnosis and prognosis of the disease, as well as the easier-to-manage diet. In general, control of blood concentrations of phe is the norm.

Russell, Mills and Zucconi (1988) reported that parents do not consider care in the first year of life to be a burden. However, they revealed that care can become incredibly difficult as children grow, due to the search for a variety of foods.

According to Castro *et al.* (2012) and Papalia and Olds (2000), dietary transgressions become more common, especially after the age of two, and can be explained by strict dietary restrictions, as well as social, cultural and behavioural factors.

Therefore, as the child grows up, he or she gains autonomy and social interaction, and difficulties in adhering to treatment arise with a progressive increase in the demands placed on families.

Carvalho (2008) and MacDonald (2010) reported in their studies that when coping with chronic illnesses, which require complex, ongoing and lifelong treatment, emotional, socioeconomic and cultural conditions must be taken into account. The authors emphasise that it is in this context that the illness emerges and it is with this socio-family structure that they will respond to this situation.

It is known that the impact of the diagnosis on the patient and their family needs to be understood, and it is thought that the disease somehow alters the social role of the sick individual. Thus, the consequences of PKU extend to the family structure, imposing the need to reorganise in order to meet daily demands and care for dietary treatment.

The experience acquired over more than twenty years of running the SR shows the importance of the social implications of PKU treatment, which mainly affect the family dealing with a special diet, since it is extremely restrictive and different from the cultural habits of the Brazilian population, instituted when the disease is diagnosed and which must be maintained for life.

The author of this study has been observing the work process at the Phenylketonuria Outpatient Clinic for sixteen years as a nutritionist at PETN-MG. It was from this context, following the various difficulties faced by families, from diagnosis to treatment of PKU, that the question arose:

- How does Phenylketonuria affect the life of the child and the family?

According to Turato, Fontanella and Campos (2006), broadening scientific understanding of phenomena about life and illness, such as those experienced and symbolised by patients and their families, are needs that health professionals often face. Based on the premise that the former have life experiences and specific information that will help them understand various health and life problems, these professionals take on the specific role of clinical investigator.

Perriconi *et al.* (2013) in their study concluded that mothers' coping skills in response to chronic illness (CD) can enable the healthcare team involved in a child's care not only to understand how parents cope with a distressing event, but also to provide them with the necessary professional support.

Burgard (2007) revealed that it is up to the health care team that treats phenylketonurics to understand the difficulties of dealing with a chronic condition and its impact on daily life. Patients and their families need to be supported, not blamed, and health professionals need to be trained in adherence in order to become skilled at listening differently to the difficulties presented. It is therefore essential for the team to identify treatment challenges and propose strategies to overcome them. In this way, it will be possible to direct the team's intervention, aiming for responses that take into account singular demands, because the experience of illness is unique for each user and their family. They must be recognised by health professionals as active social actors, participants and co-responsible in the treatment process, respecting their emotional, social, economic and cultural difficulties that impose limits on coping with PKU.

At a time when the country is taking a clear direction in favour of policies committed to improving the population's living conditions, health policies must contribute by carrying out the task of producing health and subjects in an attuned way, in the fight to guarantee ethical principles in dealing with human life (BRASIL, 2011).

It is important to emphasise that the treatment of PKU is complex and at the same time effective, and is carried out entirely by the SUS. The flow through the public health network is established from neonatal screening and diagnosis, to treatment, the release of special formula for PKU and care by a multidisciplinary team.

The National Policy for the Humanisation of SUS Care and Management is committed to the inseparability between ways of producing health and ways of managing work processes, between care and management; between clinical practice and politics; between the production of health and the production of subjectivity. Operating on the principle of transversality, HumanizaSUS uses tools to consolidate networks, links and co-responsibility between users, workers and managers. By directing strategies and methods for articulating actions, knowledge and subjects, it is possible to effectively enhance the guarantee of comprehensive, resolutive and humanised care (BRASIL, 2011).

According to Waldow and Borges (2011), care and humanisation have been the subject of great interest in the health area and the former is often referred to as secondary to humanisation. However, care is the category that characterises the humanness of being. Care is an ethical ideal; it can be nurtured, developed and its fundamental aspect is the shift of interest from our reality to that of the other. According to the authors, compassion, competence, trust, awareness and commitment are basic caring behaviours. Care, therefore, involves acts, behaviours and attitudes. Adopting the category of care, instead of humanisation, allows us to see the human being in a more complete, integral way and, considering their ontological and existential bases, as a unique, singular and unrepeatable being. Thus, care becomes an exercise; it is what the professional will add to their actions, unleashing the process of caring, which is coated with their own knowledge, sensitivity, intuition and moral values and principles. Humanising healthcare involves respecting the uniqueness of each person, personalising care and should not be seen as something that can be trained, but rather sensitised (WALDOW; BORGES, 2011).

Humanising health care and management in the SUS is an unequivocal strategy that effectively contributes to the qualification of comprehensive, equitable care, with accountability and bonds. It can be said that the Health Humanisation Network is a network for permanently building bonds of citizenship. It is therefore about looking at each individual in their specificity, their life story, encouraging them to take a leading role in the health system (BRASIL, 2011).

One of the guidelines of the National Humanisation Policy is the *Expanded and Shared Clinic*, which aims to improve the way health is done. The expanded clinic works on the harms and benefits generated by health practices, and relies on teams from different specialities sharing responsibility with users and their surroundings (BRASIL, 2009).

Thus, understanding the precepts of the SUS, this study starts from the premise that the aggregation of knowledge between professionals, patients and families promotes humanised care in PKU, highlighting the importance of reinforcing the concept of humanisation defended by the public health service.

In qualitative research it is also essential to specify the working hypothesis, as a reconstructive roadmap, openly directed, to build theoretical bases and select relevance (DEMO, 1998).

This study hypothesises that PKU, like other chronic diseases, causes disorganisation in family dynamics with psychological, behavioural, social, economic and cultural repercussions, significantly affecting the affected individual in their environment.

The scientific literature presents various studies on PKU, but little has been done on the repercussions of diagnosis and living with the disease. Considering that there are a significant number of PKU patients in the state of Minas Gerais when compared to other care centres around the world, the importance of carrying out research of this nature is confirmed.

The study was proposed on the basis of initial questions, recognising the importance of broadening the understanding of the aspects involved in the treatment of PKU, beyond purely biological issues. Its aims are to understand the mother's perception of the repercussions of PKU on family dynamics and the perception of the multi-professional team on the care and treatment of the affected child, with a view to improving the care and quality of life of phenylketonurics and their families.

> *"On our journey, sharing breaks down barriers,*
> *creates bonds, builds unity and solidarity."*
> *(Fr Nilo Luza)*

CHAPTER 2

Phenylketonuria: a literature review

"When you think you've arrived, you discover
that you have to go further. One road ends,
another begins. The immensity of life will
always be in front of us, ready to be lived as
many times as necessary."
(Message of Light and Peace)

Concept and diagnosis

Phenylketonuria (PKU) is an autosomal recessive genetic disease caused by a mutation in a gene that codes for the enzyme phenylalanine hydroxylase (PHA) located on the long arm of chromosome twelve (SCRIVER; KAUFMAN, 2001). It is the most frequent of the metabolic diseases and the most serious of the hyperphenylalaninemias (HPA), and is present in various ethnic groups, with a varied incidence. The global average is one positive case for every 11,000 live births (1:11,000), and in Brazil the incidence is 1:22,000 (BRASIL, 2012).

There are several types of PAH, and in the classic form, called PKU, the enzymatic activity of PHA is absent or less than 2% (MIRA; MARQUEZ, 2000; STARLING *et al*, 1999). Generally speaking, PAHs are defined by blood concentrations of phe above 240 pmol/L (SCRIVER; KAUFMAN, 2001). The transient form, in general, is due to the immaturity of the liver in pre-term and malnourished newborns in the womb, or to feeding errors due to excessive protein intake in the neonatal period. In this case, the

phe concentrations normalise by the age of six months (SCRIVER; KAUFMAN, 2001; SMITH; LEE, 2000).

Continuously high concentrations of phe in the blood characterise persistent HPA, which is genetic in origin and is most often caused by an absence or deficiency in the activity of the enzyme PHA, which is responsible for hydroxylating phe into tyrosine (tyr). Tetrahydrobiopterin Deficiency (BH4) is another group of HPA, consisting of a defect in the BH4 cofactor. Previously, it was described as malignant Phenylketonuria, because it did not respond to dietary treatment and therefore diet alone did not prevent the general delay in neuropsychomotor development (SULLIVAN; CHANG, 1999). Deficiency of the enzyme or a defect in its cofactor BH4 causes an increase in L-phe and its secondary metabolites in the blood and tissues, leading to the main signs and symptoms of the disease, which can manifest themselves to a greater or lesser extent (MARTINS *et aL,* 2006; SCRIVER; KAUFMAN, 2001; SURTEES; BLAU, 2000).

According to residual enzyme activity, persistent PAH can be classified into two different forms: Benign PAH (non-phenylketonuric or permanent) and classical phenylketonuria, also known as PKU. In the benign form, PHA activity is higher than 5% of what is expected and blood concentrations of phe remain between 240 pmol/L and 600 pmol/L (> 4 mg/dL and < 10 mg/dL), with the usual diet without any restrictions (SMITH; LEE, 2000). In PKU, blood concentrations of phe are higher than 600 pmol/L (10 mg/dL). In an attempt to excrete the excess phe from the blood, a second pathway of metabolism is activated, resulting in high concentrations, not only of the amino acid, but also of its metabolites in the blood and other body fluids, the cerebrospinal fluid in particular.

According to Smith and Lee (2000), excess phe and its catabolites have a toxic effect on somatic and central nervous system functions, interfering with brain protein synthesis and myelination, reducing the formation of serotonin and altering the concentration of amino acids in the cerebrospinal fluid. The authors also reported that chronically high concentrations of phe can inhibit the transport of other amino acids to the brain, especially tyrosine and tryptophan, through competition. This inhibition can occur through both the blood-brain barrier and the neuronal cytoplasmic membrane, resulting in reduced synthesis of proteins and neurotransmitters.

PKU should preferably be diagnosed in the neonatal period, before clinical symptoms appear, as the neurological damage is irreversible. The neonatal screening test, carried out between the third and fifth day of the baby's life, makes it possible to identify the individual with a suspected diagnosis and provide early treatment. Newborns who present blood phe concentrations below 240 pmol/L during neonatal screening are considered normal. Those with results between 240 pmol/L and 600 pmol/L repeat the screening test and, if the result is still above 240 pmol/L, are referred for a first consultation. Newborns whose first screening test results are above 600 pmol/L are immediately referred for a first consultation (STARLING *etal.*, 1999).

Depending on the results of the examination at the start of treatment, the initial diagnosis is established and the specific course of action is defined, as shown in Table 2.1.

Table 2.1 **Phenylalanine blood concentrations, probable diagnoses and recommended behaviour at the first consultation**

Phe dosage	Probable diagnosis	Behaviour
< 240 µmol/L (< 4 mg/dL)	Transient hyperphenylalaninaemia (HPT)	Follow-up for 6 months. If blood concentrations of phe are maintained without dietary restrictions, the child is discharged from the service.
≥ 240 µmol/L and < 600 µmol/L (≥ 4 mg/dL and < 10 mg/dL)	Benign Hyperphenylalaninaemia (HPP)	Adequacy of the diet in terms of the amount of protein and monitoring of the child until the age of 6, when they will be discharged from the service. The girl is recommended to return to the clinic in her early teens[1] .
phe ≥ 600 µmol/L (≥ 10 mg/dL)	Phenylketonuria	Immediate dietary treatment.

Source: **Starling et al., 1999.**

[1]Girls in the period of puberty are advised to return to the clinic for follow-up and dietary advice, due to the potential risk of teratogenicity from high blood concentrations of phe.

Clinical aspects

Children with PKU have no apparent abnormalities at birth, as the mother's liver protects the foetus. The blood levels of phe in phenylketonuric newborns increase in the first few weeks with protein feeding, including breast milk (MONTEIRO; CÂNDIDO, 2006).

Persistent elevations in blood concentrations of phe and its metabolites can reach levels ten to twenty times higher than normal, producing toxic effects on the central nervous system. Children are unable to reach normal developmental milestones, as neurological lesions, which are not present at birth, progressively compromise brain function with the development of mental retardation (NATIONAL INSTITUTES OF HEALTH, 2001; MONTEIRO; CÂNDIDO, 2006; SULLIVAN; CHANG, 1999).

Affected individuals without early diagnosis and treatment develop clinical manifestations in the first months of life (between the third and sixth month). These include protein-energy malnutrition, eczema, a characteristic smell (of mould or rats) in the urine, hyperactivity, hyper-reflexia, convulsions, microcephaly, autistic behaviour, motor and behavioural disorders, language delay and neuropsychomotor development in general with mental retardation of varying intensity, but always irreversible (ACOSTA; YANNICELLI, 2001; CLARK, 1992; SCRIVER; KAUFMAN, 2001; SURTEES; BLAU, 2000).

Inadequate control of blood concentrations of phe leads to metabolic alterations with low concentrations of adrenaline, dopamine, noradrenaline and serotonin. These alterations cause phenylketonurics to lose their functions, especially their intellectual capacity. It is estimated that a patient can lose an average of five Intelligence Quotient (IQ) units for every 10 weeks of delay in treatment. In addition to the reduction in intellectual quotient, it can cause slow thinking, learning difficulties, anxiety and personality disorders (MONTEIRO; CÂNDIDO, 2006; MIRA; MARQUEZ, 2000).

Researchers interested in understanding the mechanisms that cause brain damage in PKU patients with early treatment have sought to establish associations between blood Phe concentrations and intellectual performance (SCHWEITZER-KRANTZ; BURGARD, 2000).

It should also be emphasised that PKU patients have blood concentrations of phe two to ten times higher than non-phenylketonuric individuals. This effect of the disease occurs even in patients with early diagnosis and good treatment control (HUIJBREGTS *et al,* 2002). Thus, the quality of treatment control is yet another factor to be considered. The higher the levels of blood phe, the greater the amount of body phe, which can represent a greater amount of brain phe, thus interfering with the Central Nervous System, depending on the activity of the blood-brain barrier (PIETZ *et aL,* 2002).

National Neonatal Screening Programme

Screening for diseases, using complementary tests in the immediate period or close to birth, is now internationally widespread as a relevant public health practice. However, no matter how sensitive and specific the laboratory screening method is, the final diagnosis is eminently clinical and depends on additional tests to confirm the initial suspicion (JANUÁRIO, 2013).

In Brazil, the Statute of the Child and Adolescent, Federal Law No. 8069, of 13 July 1990, made it compulsory for hospitals and other health care establishments for pregnant women, both public and private, to carry out tests aimed at diagnosing and treating abnormalities in the newborn's metabolism, as well as providing guidance to the parents on any diseases diagnosed (BRASIL, 1990). Since then, some states have set up Newborn Screening Programmes. Between 1992 and 1993, the State Health Departments took over these programmes (MONTEIRO; CÂNDIDO, 2006).

The Minas Gerais State Neonatal Screening Programme (PETN-MG) was created in 1993 and is coordinated by the State Health Department. The Centre for Action and Research in Diagnostic Support at the UFMG Faculty of Medicine (NUPAD-FM-UFMG) is the programme's executing body, responsible for the treatment and laboratory tests carried out in the state's 853 municipalities to screen for Phenylketonuria, congenital hypothyroidism, sickle cell anaemia, cystic fibrosis, biotinidase deficiency and congenital adrenal hyperplasia.

The experiences of neonatal screening programmes show important data, such as the possibility of coverage with quality and agility, integrating the basic health network with the reference centre (HOROVITZ; LLERENA JR.; MATTOS, 2005).

The National Newborn Screening Programme (PNTN) was an initiative of the Ministry of Health, with the aim of implementing and regulating Newborn Screening in Brazil. On 6th June 2001, Ministry of Health (MOH) Ordinance GM/MS No. 822 triggered this process, transforming the Newborn Screening (NT) test into a Programme with emphasis on all stages, from sample collection to treatment and follow-up of patients by a multidisciplinary team. The PNTN brought a new perspective to NB in the public health system, which has remained the same to this day. Some of the actions implemented stand out:

- reinforced compulsory screening for Phenylketonuria (PKU) and Congenital Hypothyroidism, and included screening for Sickle Cell Disease/other Haemoglobinopathies and for Cystic Fibrosis;
- accredited management and assistance units in each state, the

Reference Services in Neonatal Screening (SRTN), which have a multidisciplinary team including a nutritionist trained in the care of phenylketonurics;

- has made amino acid formula for phenylketonurics available through the State Health Departments, as well as essential medicines for the treatment of patients detected with the four diseases screened in the programme;
- has provided important official data and can be considered a successful public health programme. In eleven years, the PNTN has screened more than twenty million newborns in the twenty-seven (27) Federative Units and thirty (30) SRTN, achieving a coverage rate of around 80 per cent of Brazilian live births (BRASIL, 2012).

In Minas Gerais, neonatal screening covers 100 per cent of the municipalities in the state, covering approximately 94 per cent of the state's live births. PKU has an incidence of one case for every 21,175 live births screened. Considering that NUPAD carries out an average of 22,000 tests a month, it is expected that a new patient will be identified every month and begin treatment (AGUIAR, 2004; MARTINS, 2005).

NT does not end with the results of the tests, and various actions must be taken to treat and monitor affected children, since they are subject to irreversible damage to their growth and development, and may even die early (JANUÁRIO, 2013).

Clinical-nutritional monitoring of PKU patients in the state of Minas Gerais is centralised in Belo Horizonte at the Phenylketonuria Outpatient Clinic of the Special Genetics Service of the Hospital das Clínicas of the Federal University of Minas Gerais (SEG-HC-UFMG). NUPAD has a team of doctors, nutritionists, psychologists, nurses and social workers, working in an integrated way to provide care and support for all PKU patients undergoing treatment. It also relies on the activities of the Education and Social Support Centre (CEAPS) and the Treatment Control Sector (SCT), which are responsible for actively seeking out and welcoming patients and their families on consultation days. Free treatment, offered by the SUS, is guaranteed to all phenylketonuric patients living in Minas Gerais, screened or not by the Programme, with early or late diagnosis (KANUFRE *et al.*, 2001a).

According to the protocol established in the state, carrying out the test from the third to the fifth day of life allows early treatment to prevent clinical manifestations of the disease. Recommending this period for the test reduces the number of false-negative cases of PKU, as well as meeting the requirement that the child be on a protein diet for at least 48 hours before the blood test (STARLING *etal.*, 1999).

Treatment

Treatment for PKU is dietary and should preferably be started by the child's twenty-first day of life (MONTEIRO; CÂNDIDO, 2006; NATIONAL INSTITUTES OF HEALTH CONSENSUS, 2001).

The diet is based on strict protein restriction and in order to achieve the recommended daily protein intake without excessive intake of phe, it is essential to use a protein substitute. This is usually an amino acid formula free of or low in phe, supplemented with tyr, selenium, vitamins and minerals. The protein substitute should preferably be used together with a natural protein, and therefore during or immediately after meals, as its absorption is compromised because it is made up exclusively of free amino acids. It is fundamental to treatment because, as well as allowing affected individuals to grow and develop properly, it also helps to stabilise blood concentrations of phe by supplying and supplementing the necessary protein intake, thus avoiding protein catabolism (BONN, 2010; MARTINS *et aL,* 1993; STARLING et a/., 2005).The blood concentrations of phe considered safe for phenylketonurics are higher than those standardised for individuals without the disease. According to Table 2.2, the SEG-HC-UFMG adopts the phe reference values recommended by the British Protocol (WAPPNER *et al.,* 1999).

Table 2.2 Recommended blood phe levels according to the patient's age

Age (years)	Blood levels of phe	
	μmol/L	mg/dL
RN a <6	≥120 ≤360	≥2≤6
≥6< 10	≥120 ≤480	≥2≤8
≥10	≥120 ≤700	≥ 2 ≤11,5

Source: **Modified from Wappner *et al.*,1999.**   NB= newborn

Until the 1980s, in all PKU treatment centres, breastfeeding was discontinued when starting the PKU diet, and a modified milk formula with a low phe content was introduced into the newborns' diet. Breast milk was not used due to the presumed difficulty of verifying the amount of phe ingested by the children and, consequently, controlling the blood levels of this amino acid. In the 1990s, a new technique was described in which the volume of breast milk ingested was estimated by the child's weight percentile. Special Phe-free formula should be given every three hours in a bottle, and breast milk offered on demand in between (GREVE *et aL,* 1994). This technique made it possible to use breast milk as a source of Phe in the treatment of phenylketonuric infants treated at the SEG/HC/UFMG from January 2000. Currently, the majority of children with PKU who start treatment at the SEG/HC/UFMG are breastfed. When this is not possible, modified powdered milk is indicated as a source of Phe in the infant's diet.

Child growth is a complex process, influenced by genetic, environmental and emotional factors. Adequate nutritional status from the beginning of life is indispensable for the child's normal growth and neuropsychomotor development. Due to the particularities of the diet for phenylketonurics, in addition to the intake of phe and tyr, calories and proteins must also be constantly monitored. The use of hypoprotein diets is contraindicated in the

treatment of PKU, as in addition to causing malnutrition, it leads to a decrease in tolerance to dietary phe, due to catabolism
endogenous protein, raising blood levels of the amino acid (ACOSTA; YANNICELLI, 2001).

The amino acid formula is responsible for providing approximately 80 per cent of the daily dietary protein for phenylketonurics. When the free amino acids present in these formulas are the main protein source, the daily protein recommendation is higher (BRASIL, 2012). For some authors, this daily supply should be 150% of the protein requirements recommended for individuals without the disease (ACOSTA; YANNICELLI, 2001; SHAW; LAWSON, 1994). Inadequate protein diets result in malnutrition and decreased dietary tolerance due to endogenous protein catabolism (ACOSTA; YANNICELLI, 2001). According to Brasil (2012), protein deficiency leads to growth deficits in children and weight loss in adults, osteopenia, a decrease in the concentration of prealbumin, hair loss and a decrease in Phe tolerance. In addition, these formulas should be offered in small portions throughout the day to avoid sudden increases in phe in the blood, increase the bioavailability of amino acids and prevent gastrointestinal symptoms, such as vomiting and diarrhoea, reported in children who ingest the formula only once or twice a day.

As it is an essential amino acid, Phe should be offered in quantities recommended for phenylketonurics and which allow for safe blood levels, according to the patient's age. Tyr should be supplemented in the diet by using a protein substitute, since its production may be compromised (ACOSTA; YANNICELLI, 2001; CORNEJO; RAIMAN, 2010; KANUFRE *et al.*, 2001a).

The special formula generally used is expensive and is guaranteed free of charge by the SUS to all patients being monitored at the SR. The average consumption per patient varies from two to eight cans per month, depending on age group.

Phe recommendations are individualised and depend on enzyme activity, age, growth rate and state of health. The dietary prescription of phe varies with individual tolerance, in relation to blood levels of phe, and according to age group, being higher in the first months of life (20 to 50 mg/kg/day), declining later as growth rate decreases.

In clinical practice, there is evidence of rigorous treatment due to the metabolic changes that require immediate and constant adjustments to the dietary prescription. According to the SR protocol, consultations and laboratory tests should take place weekly in the first six months of life; fortnightly from six months to one year and monthly from one to two years of age. From the age of two, consultations take place every two months, and blood samples are taken monthly, alternately in the municipality of origin and in the SR on the day of the consultation.

At six months, all patients suspected of having PKU undergo an overload test to confirm and classify the diagnosis as to the type of hyperphenylalaninaemia, as described in Table 2.3. This test consists of offering 180 mg of phe/day for three days, a concentration approximately four times higher than the recommended daily intake at this age, introducing cow's milk as a substitute for infant formula.

Table 2.3 **Classification of hyperphenylalaninemia according to the results of the overload test**

Classification/Diagnosis	Dosage of phe in the blood (pmol/L)
Classic Phenylketonuria	≥ 1200
Mild Phenylketonuria	$\geq 600 < 1200$
Permanent hyperphenylalaninaemia	$\geq 240 < 600$
Transient hyperphenylalaninaemia	< 240

Source: **Starling et al., 1999.**

a

The foods banned for PKU are those that contain a high content of proteine and, consequently, phe. These include all meats, sausages, milk and dairy products (cheese, cottage cheese, yoghurt, fakult®, Danoninho®) eggs, beans, soya, peas, lentils, chickpeas, peanuts, gelatine, wheat flour, cakes, bread and biscuits in general. Industrialised foods with high levels of Phe and special-purpose foods containing aspartame are also contraindicated (KANUFRE *et al.*, 2001, 2010; MONTEIRO; CÂNDIDO, 2006).

The foods allowed in the diet of phenylketonurics are those that contain low levels of phe (from zero to 20 mg phe/100 g of food). These include honey, fruit and gum candies, fruit lollipops, fruit popsicles, candyfloss, Yutas jam, guava, manioc flour, tapioca flour, sprinkles and sago. Beverages include artificial fruit juices, aspartame-free soft drinks, currants, tea, coffee and some vanilla, strawberry and caramel creams and puddings, as well as Phe-free *milkshake* powders (KANUFRE *et al.*, 2001a, 2010; MONTEIRO; CÂNDIDO, 2006).

Foods with a medium phe content (20 to 200 mg phe/100 g of food) can be provided in the diet, according to the prescription for this amino acid. The quantities of these foods are determined by age, individual tolerance and blood levels of phe presented periodically, according to the SR protocol. These include pasta made without eggs and with special low-protein wheat flour, rice, English potato, sweet potato, baroa potato, cassava, yam, pumpkin, courgette, aubergine, beetroot, broccoli, carrot, chayote, cauliflower, jiló, okra, cabbage, green beans, tomato, cucumber, peppers, leafy greens and fruit in general (KANUFRE *et al.*, 2001a, 2010; MONTEIRO; CÂNDIDO, 2006).

Plant foods are therefore permitted, but in strictly calculated quantities, to avoid ingesting more than each patient's individual tolerance. This implies a strict individualised vegetarian diet, free of legumes and not used on demand (STARLING *et al.*, 1999). This condition makes feeding phenylketonurics a challenge for families, especially considering the cultural habits of the Brazilian population as evidenced by the consumption of rice and beans. In addition, the diet requires numerical ability to quantify the daily phe content of the foods eaten. Tables 2.4 to 2.10 show the levels of phe in foods, in household measures and in one hundred grams (100 g) of product.

Table 2.4 **Phe content in pasta, tubers and flours, in home measurements and in 100 grams of product**

MASSES	1 tablespoonful		1 shallow tablespoon		100 grams phe (mg)
	grams	phe (mg)	grams	phe (mg)	
Boiled rice	25	27,5	15	16,5	110
Angu	35	57,8	25	41,3	165
Oats (flour)	18	125,6	8	55,8	698
Boiled potatoes	35	11,4	25	8,1	33
Boiled sweet potato	42	35,3	30	25,2	84
Sweet potato fries	65	130,0	55	110,0	200
Boiled English potato	30	26,4	20	17,6	88
English fries	25	46,0	15	27,6	184
Cassava flour	16	7,2	12	5,4	45
Boiled yams	35	25,2	22	15,8	72
Noodles without boiled eggs	25	41,5	20	33,2	166
Boiled egg noodles	25	59,0	20	47,2	236
Cooked Rilla® noodles	25	9,5	20	7,6	38
Boiled cassava	30	9,2	20	6,1	31
Fried cassava	35	21,4	20	12,2	61

Source: **Adapted from Starling *etal.*, 2006**

Table 2.5 **Phe content in type A vegetables, in homemade measures and in 100 grams of product**

VEGETABLES	1 tablespoonful		1 shallow tablespoon		100 grams phe (mg)
	grams	phe (mg)	grams	phe (mg)	
Raw chard	6	4,8	in	in	80
Lettuce	8	5,4	in	in	67
Raw leeks	10	8,0	7	5,6	80
Raw onion	10	3,8	in the	in the	38
Raw cabbage	10	4,9	7	3,4	49
Braised cabbage	20	19,6	10	9,8	98
Raw spinach	25	20,0	15	12,0	80
Sautéed spinach	25	40,0	15	24,0	160
Cucumber	18	5,4	in the	in the	30
Green chillies	13	7,0	8	4,3	54
Raw cabbage	10	5,3	5	2,6	53
Braised cabbage	18	11,3	14	8,8	63
Red tomatoes	30	6,0	20	4,0	20

Source: **Adapted from Starling *et al.*, 2006**

Table 2.6 **Phe content in type B vegetables, in homemade measures and in 100 grams of product**

TYPE B VEGETABLES	1 tablespoonful		1 shallow tablespoon		100 grams
	grams	phe (mg)	grams	phe (mg)	phe (mg)
Boiled pumpkin	36	12,4	16	5,50	34
Cooked courgette	30	24,3	20	16,2	81
Cooked aubergine	25	9,3	20	7,45	37
Raw beetroot	16	12,5	10	7,8	78
Boiled beetroot	20	9,0	14	6,3	45
Boiled broccoli	10	12,9	in	in	129
Raw carrots	12	3,7	8	2,5	31
Boiled carrots	25	9,3	15	5,6	37
Boiled chayote	20	7,4	15	5,6	37
Boiled cauliflower	25	18,7	15	11,2	75
Boiled jiló	60	40,3	30	20,2	67
Sautéed okra	40	26,8	20	13,4	67
Radish (pcs. M and P)	25	13,2	14	7,4	53
Cooked green beans	20	18,6	15	13,9	93

Source: **Adapted from Starling et al., 2006**

Table 2.7 **Phe content in fruit, in homemade measures and in 100 grams of product**

FRUIT	1 Unit/Piece* M		100 grams phe (mg)
	grams	phe (mg)	
Avocado	430	206,4	48
Pineapple	75	6,7	9
Steel	12	0,7	6
Dried black plum	5	3,9	79
Banana	40	17,6	44
Khaki	110	41,8	38
Coconut*	40	141,6	354
Coconut, water (1 American glass)	165	23,1	14
Damascus	7	2,1	30
Figs, syrup	55	18,1	33
Guava	170	42,5	25
Jaboticaba	5	1.5	30
Kiwi	76	20,5	27
Orange	180	54,0	30
Apple	150	15,0	10
Papaya Formosa*	170	22,1	13
Papaya	310	46,5	15
Mango	140	40,6	29
Passion fruit	45	29,2	65
Watermelon*	200	20,0	10
Melon*	90	15,3	17
Muskmelon	135	44,5	33
Strawberry	12	2,8	23
Pear	130	11,7	9
Peach	60	10,8	18
Grapes	8	1.2	15

Source: **Adapted from Starling *etal.*, 2006**

Table 2.8 **Phe content in canned and fatty foods, in home measurements and in 100 grams of product**

CANNED FOOD/FAT	1 tablespoonful		1 shallow tablespoon		100 grams phe (mg)
	grams	phe (mg)	grams	phe (mg)	
Green olive (un. M)	4	2,0	in the	in the	50
Black olive (un. M)	4	1,6	in the	in the	39
Green corn	24	36,0	14	in the	150
Tomato sauce	20	5,6	in the	in the	28
Peach, syrup (1/2 unit M)	30	2,7	in the	in the	9
Pineapple, syrup (1 slice M and P)	64	5,1	30	2,4	8
Pear, syrup (1 pc. M)	130	6,5	in the	in	5
Pitted plum, syrup (1 pc.)	16	1,1	in	in	7
Palm hearts (pcs. M)	100	80,0	in the	in the	80
Fresh cream	25	30,0	15	18	120
Hellmann's® mayonnaise	27	9,4	17	5,9	35
Butter	32	11,2	19	6,6	35
Margarine	32	4,5	19	2,7	14

Source: **Adapted from Starling et al., 2006**

Table 2.9 **Phe content in biscuits, bread and popcorn, in home measurements and in 100 grams of product**

BISCUITS	Average Unit		100 grams phe (mg)
	grams	phe (mg)	
Sprinkle biscuit without eggs	3	4,1	135
Sprinkle biscuits with eggs	3	6,7	225
Strawberry wafer	9	25,2	280
Chocolate wafer	9	45,8	509
Water and salt biscuit	5	22,5	450
María/Maisena biscuit	5	23,2	465
French bread	50	235,0	470
Sweet popcorn	20	99,0	495
Salted popcorn	20	139,6	698
Seven Boys® Sequilhos	3	5,6	167

Source: **Adapted from Starling *et al.*, 2006**

Table 2.10 **Phe content in other foods, per 100 grams of product**

FOOD	phe (mg)
Arisco® bean stock	350
Sugarcane juice	12
Cocoa powder	1050
Shredded coconut	270
Defatted cocoa powder	1250
Beef	910-1795
Chicken meat	880-1670
Pork	695-1725

Pea pods	375
Wheat flour	577
Soya flour	1800
Arrowroot starch	20
Arrowroot flour	70
Fresh yeast	500
Carioca beans	240
Black beans	225
Purple beans	285
Cornflour	384
Cassava flour	52
Rice starch	50
Potato starch	50
Glória® condensed milk	380
Cow's milk	170
Coconut milk	30
Lentils	315
Quail egg	655
Chicken egg	739
Fish	950-1825
Arrowroot starch	40
Rapadura	33
Siriguela	27
Umbu	18

Source: **ENDEF-IBGE, 1999; TACO, 2006**

Control and adherence to treatment should be monitored by the results of frequent blood samples, according to the protocol practised in the SR, and by evaluating the seventy-two-hour dietary records. The difficulty in adhering to the diet seems to be related to the ban on the consumption of natural proteins and the requirement to use a protein substitute, generally based on free amino acid formulas with a characteristic odour and taste, which is not very palatable and reflects a stigma for phenylketonurics.

For Garcia and Canesqui (2005), the way we eat has a greater meaning than the simple act of eating and is linked to identity and other social dimensions. Since food is shaped by culture and suffers the effects of the organisation of society, it cannot be approached unilaterally. The interaction between the cognitive and emotional dimensions involved in this behaviour is therefore evident (TORAL; SLATER, 2007).

The relationship between diet and quality of life has been intensely proven and discussed in the literature. Thus, reflection on the various aspects involved in the field of nutrition requires a shift in focus from measurable phenomena to social, psychological and cultural issues (BOOG, 1999, 2005).

The study of eating behaviour has aroused great interest because it is an important element in the success of nutritional interventions and because of the possibility of increasing the effectiveness of these interventions. Since all these factors interfere with individuals' eating behaviour, the patient's life problems need to be known and understood by the professionals who treat them (BOOG, 1997, 2008).

Araújo *et al.* (2010) reported that eating practices are social practices rooted in culture. Individuals' tastes, choices and preferences, apparently voluntary, are symbolically constructed as signs of social position, *status and* distinction. In this way, lifestyle is closely related to social position and is reflected in the choice of diet and aesthetic standards.

Treatments based on restrictive diets are related to difficulties that are exacerbated by the social and cultural nature of food. Scientific knowledge is not enough to change eating habits, because they are not based solely on human rationality or medical materialism. However, they coexist tensely with the symbolic values and pleasures provided by food, be they gustatory, psychological or social, stemming from the situations created around meals (ROMANELLI, 2006).

Simply passing on nutritional information is not enough to help patients who need to make changes to their diet, as this information only reaches the intellectual dimension and eating involves much more than that. The great challenge facing nutritional education is the need to develop educational strategies that, as well as transmitting information, enable the creation of new meanings for the act of eating (RODRIGUES; BOOG, 2005).

Nutritional education should focus on the formation of values, pleasure and responsibility, but also on play and freedom. Interdisciplinary approaches emerge as options that can offer alternative paths for this practice (BOOG, 2008). According to Freire (2003), it is important to recognise that educating is not simply transferring knowledge, but creating possibilities for its production or construction.

Araújo *et al.* (2010) reported that, in studies carried out with coeliac patients, the majority of patients interviewed revealed that they had great difficulties in choosing components of their diet. Among the problems cited were difficulties in determining whether foods were gluten-free and finding gluten-free products on the market. For these patients, situations such as travelling, eating out and socialising with friends and family can pose problems and thus interfere with their social life.

The study carried out by Di Ciommo *et al.* (2012) explored the experiences of twenty PKU patients over the age of seven, from their own point of view, mainly addressing the limitations and social stigmas arising from the diet. In this study, only one ten-year-old boy referred to Phenylketonuria as a disease; most preferred terms such as tolerance, allergy or problem. One of them revealed that it was an allergy, because there is illness when you feel ill. For him, an allergy is when you can't eat something. Eating a special food makes young people feel different. This difference was reported by the teenagers as a feeling of inferiority, discrimination and fear, at a time when they are being compared to others. Many forgo outings, school trips and parties for fear of feeling ashamed. In this specific case, the authors suggest that interventions be carried out to minimise the burden of the disease with a view to reducing its stigma and improving social adaptation.

Currently, dietary treatment is recommended throughout life, since even after the individual has fully developed neurologically, high levels of phe can alter cognitive functions. Interrupting the diet is also associated with a worsening of QoL in children and a decrease in attention and information processing speed in adults (NATIONAL INSTITUTES OF HEALTH, 2001).

Thus, patients with poor control of blood levels of Phe or who abandon treatment are subject to serious consequences, not only in terms of intellectual development, but also damage to social interaction, due to emotional instability, irritability, aggressiveness, hyperactivity, among others. The literature also describes low autonomy, low self-esteem, loneliness and sadness (SULLIVAN; CHANG, 1999; WEGLAGE; RUPP; SCHMIDT, 1994).

It should also be emphasised that a permanent and continuous diet is essential for female phenylketonurics in order to avoid maternal PKU. Children born to mothers with PKU or non-phenylketonuric hyperphenylalaninaemia who have blood phe above 240 pmol/L (4 mg/dL) are subject to low birth weight, microcephaly, mental retardation, postnatal growth retardation and congenital heart disease of varying complexity, as well as other anomalies related to the teratogenicity of high phe levels (WAISBREN *et al.*, 1997). It is therefore recommended that these patients maintain blood levels of phe below this value at least three months before conception and throughout pregnancy (BRASIL, 2012).

Since the main aspect of PKU treatment concerns diet, its

effectiveness depends largely on the extent to which the patient or their carer follows the nutritional recommendations. However, adequate engagement is not easily achieved among phenylketonurics. In the Phenylketonuria Outpatient Clinic at SEG-HC- UFMG, it has been noted that after the second year of life, dietary control and, consequently, control of blood levels of Phe, makes treatment more difficult and complex. During this period, there is a change in the consistency of the diet, greater autonomy on the part of the child due to the search for their own food, as well as an increase in social contacts in the environment in which they live, such as joining the school, visiting relatives and friends, travelling, etc. Thus, dietary transgressions become increasingly common with advancing age and can be explained by strict dietary restrictions, social, cultural and behavioural factors. As a result, the demands placed on families increase progressively.

Frank; Fitzgerald and Legge (2007) reported that adherence to treatment seems to decrease with age and that recent research shows the possibility of problems linked to cognitive aspects and social functions in adults with PKU who have discontinued dietary treatment.

However, patients' adherence to treatment and their response should not be measured solely by the blood levels of phe assessed at outpatient appointments. It is known that there is a natural tendency for human beings to seek better control and adherence to treatment in the days leading up to appointments. The biggest challenge, of course, is maintaining adequate blood control and a restrictive diet at all times.

CHAPTER 3

Chronic illness and its implications

Scientific and technological development has made it possible to diagnose diseases at an early stage, and appropriate therapy often makes it possible to control their progression and cure them. Even with these advances, some diseases, especially chronic ones, trigger organic, emotional and social changes that require constant care and adaptation. A chronic illness (CD) is one that has a long course with the possibility of sequelae, which imposes limitations on the individual's functions, requires adaptation and affects the daily lives of all family members. CD is characterised by the need for ongoing management and care, as well as follow-up by health professionals (SILVA *et al.*, 2010; VIEIRA; LIMA, 2002).

Realising the existence of the disease brings a lot of suffering for all family members and the fragility imposed by the diagnosis can lead to social exclusion, as they have to face a society that is exclusionary towards the most vulnerable (CARVALHO, 2008). According to Castro and Piccinini (2002), the social isolation of the family that has a CD patient with various restrictions is a frequent occurrence that can leave the patient more vulnerable to emotional disorders, the creation of problems in coping with the illness, as well as perpetuating the stigma.

The implications of chronic illnesses do not belong exclusively to the sick individual, but also to family members and social circles. These shared meanings, either directly or indirectly, end up influencing the evolution of the illness. They can help to reduce or increase symptoms, exaggerate or reduce difficulties, or even hinder or facilitate treatment (FERREIRA *et al.*, 2012).

(2012) and Silva *et al.* (2010), CD brings with it not only negative aspects, but also positive ones that apply even to the carer, and not just to the patient. The impact it has on the patient's family carer is important in the patient-disease relationship and is generally overlooked in clinical practice. Broadening our understanding of the experience and aspects resulting from contact with the illness is a possibility for caring: caring for the chronically ill and their family members.

It is known that CD goes beyond the limits of the child's body and affects the entire family structure, disrupting routines and emotionally shaking all its members. Faced with these situations, a multi-professional approach is essential, involving not only the clinical aspects, but also the psychological and social repercussions for both the child and the family. It is necessary for health professionals to be attentive to aspects that transcend medical treatment, because without a comprehensive view of the child's progress and relationships with those around them, the success of the treatment may be compromised (SILVA *et al.*, 2010).

The difficulties related to the nature of the treatment are evident, resulting, among other problems, in low engagement rates among patients and their families. However, despite the difficulties experienced by many families with a child with CD, some manage to make internal and external resources available and create effective strategies for dealing with the disease (SANTOS, 1998).

The adjustment of CD to the family situation is different in type and intensity depending on the stage of the life cycle the family is in. Encouraging families to anticipate problems, mobilise resources and share personal feelings encourages mother-caregivers in their caring skills (FERREIRA *et aL,* 2012).

Phenylketonuria as a chronic disease

PKU significantly affects families who will need support to adjust to the new demands. In addition to treatment based on a very restrictive diet, different from that consumed by the general population, it also requires frequent blood tests. The identification of a child with PKU can also affect their siblings, who may feel their parents' attention is more focussed on the phenylketonuric (SCHILD, 1972).

Although there are few studies dealing with the mother-child relationship with CD, the evidence shows that family relationships are fundamental to coping adequately with the disease and prolonged treatment. It can be seen that the involvement of the people who make up the social and emotional bonds of phenylketonurics can facilitate adherence to treatment, and the psychological aspects of the patient can interfere with the results. In addition, the contextualisation of family stress associated with CD, especially parental stress, needs to take into account the very characteristics of mothers and fathers, as well as their perception of their child's illness. Most children perceive the disease as something external to them, show no signs of understanding their role in treatment and believe that they will be cured in a short space of time. And the way the illness is represented by the individual influences the way they act towards it (CASTRO; PICCININI, 2002).

In short, families who experience childhood CD go through a process of reorganising their daily lives, and the health team's perception of the unique care demands of these families helps them to recognise the difficulties experienced and mobilise resources to cope and adapt (SILVA *et al.* 2010).

CHAPTER 4

Purpose of the study

> *"The art of listening is like a*
> *light that dispels the darkness*
> *of ignorance."*
> *(Dalai Lama)*

To understand the mother's perception of the repercussions of Phenylketonuria on family dynamics and the perception of the multi-professional team on care and treatment.

Step 1

To understand the mother's perception of the repercussions of Phenylketonuria on family dynamics.

- getting to know the mothers interviewed and their children with Phenylketonuria;
- understand maternal reactions to diagnosis and treatment;
- identify strategies that families and children develop to deal with the disease.

Stage 2

To understand the perception of the multi-professional team on the care and treatment of Phenylketonuria.

- learn about the difficulties and challenges encountered by the team during treatment;
- to identify the professionals' strategies for overcoming the difficulties experienced by the team;

- to subsidise team reflection in order to suggest actions to help improve adherence to treatment for Phenylketonuria.

CHAPTER 5

Methodological approach

The contribution of the social sciences to understanding behaviours linked to health and illness has been considered increasingly essential for the appropriate development of prevention and treatment actions (BOOG, 2005).

This study uses qualitative research as its methodological reference, as it is considered the most appropriate for understanding the subjective aspects of human psychosocial phenomena, including illness experiences (TOMAZI; YAMAMOTO, 1999).

This type of research seeks to interpret what people say about a phenomenon and what they do or how they deal with it. Its aim is to apprehend this knowledge from the perspective of the subject, i.e. what is manifested or perceived by their consciousness or senses and their meanings, since they constitute the core of this type of research. The researcher respects the position of the subjects being investigated, with fidelity to their speech, interpreting the results and taking into account the relationships of meaning they establish. As a result, this makes it possible to generate original knowledge (TURATO, 2003).

Sampling

In qualitative research, various sources of information must be used as a way of grasping all the elements needed to delve deeper into the reality under study.

Sampling strategies should always be determined by the purpose of the study design. Statistical representativeness is not usually sought in qualitative research. Similarly, the size of the sample is not determined by inflexible rules, but by other factors, such as the depth and duration required for each interview and the possibility of having a single interviewee (POPE; MAYS, 2006).

According to Minayo *etal.* (1994), an ideal sample is one that is capable of reflecting the whole in its multiple dimensions. Based on this, the author proposes some basic criteria for sampling:

- clearly define the most relevant social group for the interviews;
- not be exhausted until the empirical framework of the research is delineated;
- foresee a process of progressive inclusion guided by the discoveries of the field and their confrontation with theory;
- predict a triangulation.

Saturation sampling is a conceptual tool often used in qualitative research reports in different areas of the health field. It is used to establish or close the final size of a sample under study by stopping the capture of new components. The finding of saturation depends on the researcher's objectives. If the aim is to capture what characterises the group, sample saturation will occur at a certain level. This level can guarantee greater external validity, i.e. greater ability to reproduce interpretations for wider contexts (FONTANELLA; RICAS; TURATO, 2008).

The assessment of theoretical saturation from a group of

participants is made through a continuous process of analysing the data, starting at the beginning of the collection process. In view of the questions put to the interviewees, which reflect the research objectives, this preliminary analysis looks for the moment when little substantially new appears, considering each of the topics covered or identified during the analysis and the group of interviewees (FONTANELLA; RICAS; TURATO, 2008).

Data collection

The selection of the data collection instrument must take into account the objectives of the study and the most appropriate way to respond to them. As the data is collected, the researcher tries to identify themes and relationships, constructs interpretations, generates new questions or refines previous ones, which in turn leads them to look for new, complementary or more specific data to test their interpretations, in a process of fine tuning that leads up to the final analysis. Organising the data is a continuous process in which we try to identify dimensions, categories, trends, patterns and relationships, revealing their meaning. The process that accompanies all research is complex, non-linear and involves synthesising, organising and interpreting the data (ALVES-MAZZOTI et al, 2004).

Since this study was carried out in two stages, the sampling and data collection for each stage has been described separately.

Stage One: The mother's perception of the repercussions of Phenylketonuria on family dynamics

At this stage of the study, the semi-structured interview was the main instrument for data collection, since the aim was to study in depth the mother's perception of PKU in the family dynamic. The clinical and sociodemographic questionnaire was used as a complementary tool to better understand the reality under investigation.

The interview is the most commonly used qualitative technique in healthcare establishments, as it makes important contributions to obtaining not only objective but also subjective data that can reveal aspects investigated in depth (POPE; MAYS, 2006; TURATO; FONTANELLA; CAMPOS, 2006).

According to Simioni; Lefèvre; Pereira (1996) and Trivinos (1994), before starting the interview, the researcher must be fully convinced of the need to develop a climate of empathy and trust between the interviewer and the interviewee, so that the latter can speak freely about the proposed topics.

In semi-structured interviews, the interviewer does not need to ask many questions. It is recommended to use a pre-prepared script of essential questions to be addressed. This script is an instrument to guide the interview, *a conversation with a purpose,* thus allowing dialogue between interviewer and interviewee, so that it can facilitate opening up, broadening and deepening communication. In this way, the researcher invites the interviewees to talk about their own problems, interests, concerns, opinions, expectations and fears, with the aim of grasping all the ideas, feelings and attitudes of the social actors, as provided for in the study's objective (MINAYO, 2004).

Approaching individuals through semi-structured interviews implies intervening carefully in order to get as much in-depth information about their points of view as possible. Individuals are allowed to talk about the desired topics, but also about issues introduced by themselves during the interview, obviously if they are useful to the research objectives. Interviewees are expected to express themselves in their own words, behaving as an active subject in the interview. Typically, these interviews should be open-ended at the beginning, starting with a first question that is called a *trigger question.* This question focuses the research work, encouraging the generation of ideas and should be directly related to the general objective of the research. The phrase used to focus the problem should not be too general or too specific, preventing developments that are not of interest to the interviewer (TURATO; FONTANELLA; CAMPOS, 2006).

In this context, the triggering question for this study was: *How does Phenylketonuria interfere in the lives of children and their families?*

Interviews with mothers

The subjects chosen for this study were mothers of phenylketonuric children, since mothers are considered privileged informants on the health of the child, as well as representing the majority of carers who take their children to the Referral Service (RS). The inclusion criteria were: being the mother of a child aged between two and six years old, with an early diagnosis of PKU and undergoing regular treatment at the Phenylketonuria Outpatient Clinic of the Special Genetics Service of the UFMG Hospital das Clínicas (SEG-HC-UFMG). This age group was chosen because, according to the literature and the experience at SR, diet control becomes more difficult from the age of two onwards. Children experiment more, explore their environment, are more curious about what's around them and food is part of this context. These results were also found in the literature (CASTRO *et al.,* 2012; PAPALIA; OLDS, 2000).

Mothers with more than one child with PKU were excluded in order to highlight reactions to a new disease event in the family.

In order to identify eligible mothers, a search was made of the NUPAD database from 01/09/2010 until 31/03/2011, when sample saturation was reached. During this period, forty mothers met the inclusion criteria.

For data collection, the interviews were carried out in October and November 2011, based on a pre-prepared script of six questions, based on the review of related literature, the experience acquired by the researcher at the Phenylketonuria Outpatient Clinic of the SEG-HC-UFMG and in accordance with the objectives of the study. These include:

- What was it like to be told that your son had Phenylketonuria?
- What's it been like living with that?
- What has changed?
- How do you perceive your child's reaction to the diet?
- What are the biggest difficulties?
- How do you perceive the treatment and follow-up?

The mothers were recruited at the Centre for Education and Social Support (CEAPS), in the interval between the child's blood test for Phe and the appointment at the Phenylketonuria Outpatient Clinic at SEG-HC-UFMG.

After introducing the researcher, a brief explanation of the research was given and the Informed Consent Form was signed (Figure 5.1).

Figura 5.1 **Informed Consent Form (ICF) for mothers of children with PKU**

TERM OF FREE AND INFORMED CONSENT (TCLE)

Project title: "Diagnosis of Phenylketonuria: repercussions on the family and social relations".

Dear Mrs
This information letter may contain words that you do not understand. Please ask the person in charge of the study or one of the team members to explain any information that you do not clearly understand.

Purpose of the study
You are being invited to take part in a study called: "Diagnosis of Phenylketonuria: repercussions on the family and social relations".

I'm developing this project to find out about the repercussions of the diagnosis of Phenylketonuria on the family and on social relationships, through interviews with the mothers of children being treated at the Phenylketonuria Outpatient Clinic at UFMG's Hospital das Clínicas.

Those of you who have been following your child's treatment are no doubt familiar with this disease. Phenylketonuria is a hereditary disease caused by the deficiency of an enzyme produced by the liver, responsible for metabolising phenylalanine, leading to an accumulation of this substance in the blood.

Neonatal screening carried out on the 5th° day of life makes it possible to make an early diagnosis and start treatment to prevent irreversible mental retardation and the onset of the clinical manifestations of the disease, which occur from 3° to 6° months of age. Treatment is dietary and must be maintained throughout life. This can interfere with family dynamics, given the need for a very restricted diet that differs from that usually consumed in our population.

Having worked in this outpatient clinic for twelve years, I realised the need to understand how families live with the diagnosis of Phenylketonuria. The aim of this study is to investigate the repercussions of the diagnosis of Phenylketonuria on the family and social relationships, seeking to better understand the aspects that interfere with treatment, with a view to improving patient follow-up and suggesting alternatives that can help control blood levels of phenylalanine and improve the quality of life of patients and their families.

Procedures to be used
All mothers of phenylketonuric patients aged between 6 months and 6 years, with an early diagnosis and undergoing regular treatment at the Phenylketonuria Outpatient Clinic at the UFMG Hospital das Clínicas, will be invited to take part in this study.

Interviews will be held with the mothers who agree to take part in the study. The clinical-nutritional follow-up routine will be maintained as normal, according to the service's protocol, where blood is taken in the morning for phenylalanine levels and the patient is seen in the afternoon with the results of the blood test.

Your participation in the research will be voluntary and will not involve any risk for you or your child. The only possible discomfort is the length of the interview. However, the interview can be interrupted at any time if you feel the need and, if you agree, we will schedule it to continue at another time.

It is important to emphasise that there will be no compensation for participating in the research, as the interviews will take place on the same day as your child's appointment.

The results of this research will be very important and disseminated in order to understand and evaluate the aspects involved in the treatment of Phenylketonuria in our environment, improving communication

between family members and the care team, as well as identifying factors that help treatment and improve adherence to the diet.

Please note that the interviews will be recorded and/or transcribed, that all information obtained will be considered confidential and that your identification will be kept confidential. The results of this study may be presented in scientific papers and events without any form of individual identification. The identity of your child and their family will be kept confidential, as will the results of the interviews. Your participation is free and can be interrupted at any time without jeopardising your child's treatment.

If you agree to take part in this research by giving us the interview, the researcher asks you to sign this document in two copies.

Post-informed consent
I, the person responsible for the minor, _______________________________declare that I have
read (or heard) and understood what is explained in the information letter to mothers and that all
my doubts have been clarified in person.

I therefore authorise my participation in the study "Diagnosis of Phenylketonuria: repercussions
on the family and social relations". I also authorise the interviews and their use for scientific
research purposes.

I discussed my decision to take part in the research with the nutritionist in charge. It was made
clear to me what the objectives were, the procedures to be carried out, the risks, discomforts and
benefits, and the guarantees of confidentiality of my identity and that of my child.

It is also clear that my participation will be free of charge and that I will have access to the results.
I may withdraw from participation at any time during the research, without prejudice to my child's
treatment at the Phenylketonuria Outpatient Clinic at the UFMG Hospital das Clínicas.

Legible signature of the person responsible

Contact   telephone   numbers:

Note: Signed copies of the consents are kept on file by the researcher and given to the mothers
interviewed.

Signature of the researcher responsible:

Nutritionist Rosângelis Del Lama Soares - CRN/MG: 0122 CI: M2-999880

Contact telephone numbers of the researcher in charge:
(31)3285-1067 or (31) 99952-4789

If you have any questions, you can contact the researcher, Rosângelis (Tel.: 3285-1067 / 99952-
4789) or the UFMG Research Ethics Committee. Address: Av. Antônio Carlos, 6627.
Administrative Unit II, 2º floor. Pampulha Campus. BH-MG. Brazil Tel: (31) 3409-4592.

Belo Horizonte,20 _______________________________ .

Next, a questionnaire was used to characterise the mothers and their
children with PKU (Figure 5.2), including clinical and
sociodemographic information, with the aim of identifying aspects that
could contribute to understanding the reality under study.

Figura 5.2   **Clinical and sociodemographic questionnaire applied to
families of children with PKU**

CLINICAL AND SOCIODEMOGRAPHIC QUESTIONNAIRE

Diagnosis of Phenylketonuria: Repercussions on the family and social relations

Interview no.: Date: ______//
SOCIAL EVALUATION
1. IDENTIFICATION
Patient's name:No. in offspring:
Date of birth: ____// Age: _____________ Sex: Male ( ) Female ( )
Religion: ____
                    Nomedamãe :

Age:Education: (last year   )
Religion: _____________________
Municipality: Distance from BH: Km
Phone:_____________________
You live with a partner: Yes ( ) No ( ) You are the biological father: Yes ( ) No ( )
Consanguinity between parents: Yes ( ) No ( )
Do you work outside the home: Yes ( ) No ( )

Child attends school: Yes ( ) No ( ) Since what age:
Do you have any difficulties: Yes ( ) No ( )
Who looks after the child: ____

2. CLINICAL HISTORY

Age at screening test:Result of 1st[a] blood sample:pcromol/L
Result at 1[a] consultation:pcromol/L Start of treatment (age):
Overload test result:pcromol/L Diagnosis:
Average blood phe (last 6 months):pcromol/L.
Adequate: Yes ( ) No ( )
Attendance at appointments:
Dietary transgression: Yes ( ) No ( )
Quantity ( ) Quality ( ) Which: _____________________________________
Other pathologies: Yes ( ) No ( )
Which ones: ____

Use of continuous medication: Yes ( ) No ( )
Which ones: ____

3. FAMILY SITUATION (living in the same household)

Name of mum	age	Degree of kinship	Marital status	Level of education	Profession	Employment relationship	Income

Note: No. of inhabitants in the household: No. of adults:No. of children:
Other Sources of Income: Yes ( ) No ( )
Which ones:____
Are there any residents in the household with health problems: Yes ( ) No ( ) Who::

4. SOCIAL SUPPORT

Financial support: Yes ( ) No ( )
Which ones: ____
Social support: Yes ( ) No ( ) Which:_________________________________
Note: If yes, ask if it is family, third-party, institutional, municipal, other.

5. EXPENSES

Housing: R$Light: R$Water: R$
Other R$Per capita income: R$
Note ____

6. HOUSING AND HEALTH SITUATION

Housing: Owned ( ) Rented ( ) Shared ( ) With others ( )
Rural ( ) Urban ( ) Other ( ) Which:
No. of rooms without a bathroom:No. of bedrooms:Where the child sleeps:
Toilets: Yes ( ) No: Inside ( ) Outside ( ) No ( )
                        No ( )
Water supply: Mains ( ) Well ( ) Spring ( ) Other ( )
Which ones: ____
Sanitary drain: General sewage network ( ); Pit ( ); Open ground ( ); Other ( ) Waste disposal:
Collected by the municipality ( ); Burned ( );Recycled ( );Other ( ) Electricity: Yes ( ) No ( )
Vegetable garden: Yes ( ) No ( )
Is there space for cultivation: Yes ( ) No ( )

7. BASIC HEALTH UNIT

Household covered by the Family Health Programme (PSF): Yes ( ) No ( ) Does the UBS know
about your child's diagnosis (PKU): Yes ( ) No ( ) Does the PSF visit your home: Yes ( ) No ( )
How regularly:____

8. DIGITAL INCLUSION

Computer access: Yes ( ) No ( ) Internet access: Yes ( ) No ( )

9. DIFFICULTY GETTING THE TFD:
Yes ( ) No ( ) Sometimes ( )

10. TFD'S MEANS OF TRANSPORT
Ambulance ( ) Bus ( ) Own car ( ) Do you do bailing: Yes ( ) No ( ) Sometimes: ( )

All the interviews followed the pre-established script and were recorded on MP3 with the informant's authorisation. The recordings varied in length, depending on the course of the interview, from eighteen to thirty-nine minutes each. The anonymity of the participating mothers was guaranteed, and they were identified in their reports in the chronological order in which the interviews took place. Using the saturation criterion, fourteen mothers were interviewed, thus constituting the sample.

Subsequently, the interviews were transcribed in full by the researcher with the help of two undergraduate nutrition students from the Federal University of Minas Gerais, thus enabling a better understanding of the recorded content.

Stage Two: The multi-professional team's perception of the care and treatment of Phenylketonuria

Considering the objectives of the research, the Focus Group (FG) was chosen to collect data for this investigation with the participation of professionals working in the SR in the state of Minas Gerais.

The FG is one of the oral reporting strategies that values the lived experiences of the research subjects and what they have to say about them, as well as favouring communication based on a particular focus, a particular point (RIGOTTO, 1998).

Because it is relatively simple and quick, the FG has been widely used to structure public health actions. It also seems to respond well to the new trend in health education, which has shifted from the perspective of the individual to social groups, observing the cultural perspective of its potential beneficiaries. In the area of health, this is a new option, because at the same time as it allows the researcher to obtain data for their studies, it provides those being researched with a space for reflection and self-evaluation, which makes it possible to change behaviour (IERVOLINO; PELICIONI, 2001).

This technique is a type of group interview that emphasises communication between research participants, based on topics provided by the researcher. Its aim is to identify the perception of the phenomenon studied from the perspective of the actors directly involved in the issue, with the aim of generating distinct data through interaction between its members. It should be emphasised that the researcher's interest guides the focus, but the data is brought about by group interaction (KITZINGER, 2006).

Group interaction favours the disinhibition and participation of the group members, making it possible to capture the reality experienced by the participants, as well as their feelings, attitudes, ideas and information on the subject. This interaction can produce data that would be difficult to obtain outside the group (MORGAN, 1997).

Focus group with the multi-professional team

Ten professionals from different areas of knowledge who work in the reception and care of phenylketonuric patients in the SR were invited to take part in this study. The inclusion criteria were: being a professional from the Phenylketonuria Outpatient Clinic of the SEG-HC/NUPAD/FM/UFMG, the Treatment Control Sector (SCT-NUPAD) and the Education and Social Support Centre (CEAPS-NUPAD) involved in the treatment of phenylketonurics.

Two invited professionals didn't turn up for the FG activity, as previously scheduled. Eight took part, including paediatricians and geneticists, nutritionists, nurses, social workers, technicians and administrative assistants. The counsellor and the author of this research who conducted the dynamics were excluded.

For data collection, a pre-prepared script of five questions was used, based on the review of related literature, the experience acquired by the researcher at the Phenylketonuria Outpatient Clinic and in accordance with the objectives of the study. These included:

- What has it been like caring for children with Phenylketonuria and their families?
- What is your perception of approaching parents and family members at the 1ª consultation?
- How do you perceive adherence to treatment?
- From an institutional point of view, what are the biggest difficulties the service encounters and the strategies to overcome them?
- What major challenges do you identify in the treatment and follow-up of children with an early diagnosis of PKU? A few precautions were taken to ensure a relaxed atmosphere conducive to the exchange of experiences and perspectives, as guided by Morgan (1997):

- The session was held in a closed room with no noise, so there would be no interruptions.
- The chairs were arranged in a circle to encourage everyone to take part and for the participants to make good eye contact.
- The participants were explained the objectives of the meeting and the importance of speaking one at a time.
- No other participant was allowed in after the start of the session.
- Two tape recorders were used to record the speeches, reports and

discussions.

Before starting the FG activities, the researcher gave a brief explanation of the study and its objectives. The use of the recording tool, its purpose and importance were explained. The Informed Consent Form (ICF) and the Informed Consent Form (Figure 5.3) were presented to the participants and, after reading them, they signed them. The participants then introduced themselves.

The duration of the FG was one hour and eighteen minutes (1.18 hours). The entire discussion was recorded on MP3 and the audio material collected was transcribed in its entirety by the researcher with the help of an undergraduate nutrition student. The anonymity of the group members was preserved. To guarantee the confidentiality of the information, the participants were identified by codes (P1, P2, ..., P8).

Figure 5.3 **Informed Consent Form (ICF) for team members**

TERM OF FREE AND INFORMED CONSENT (TCLE)

Project title: "Diagnosis of Phenylketonuria: repercussions on the family and social relations".

Dear Sir

You are being invited to take part in the study: "Diagnosis of Phenylketonuria: repercussions on the family and social relationships".

I'm in the final phase of the project I started in 2010 on the repercussions of the diagnosis of Phenylketonuria on the family and social relationships, through interviews with the mothers of children aged 2 to 6 being treated at the Phenylketonuria Outpatient Clinic of the Special Genetics Service of the Hospital das Clínicas/ NUPAD/ FM/ UFMG.

The second phase of this project consists of investigating the perception of the multi-professional team on the impact of the diagnosis of Phenylketonuria on the family and the factors that influence treatment.

In order to achieve the proposed objective of "Understanding the perception of the multi-professional team on the factors that influence the treatment of Phenylketonuria", we opted to use the Focus Group (FG), a qualitative methodology data collection tool.

Focus groups are a type of group interview that values communication between participants in order to generate data. People are encouraged to talk to each other, exchange ideas, ask questions and comment on experiences.

Professionals from the various fields involved in the neonatal screening and treatment of Phenylketonuria and who can contribute to understanding aspects that interfere with treatment will be invited.

The meeting will take place on a single day, preferably on the same day as the weekly meeting to discuss the cases to be seen at the outpatient clinic, and will last up to 90 minutes.

The results of this research will be very important and disseminated in order to understand and evaluate the aspects involved in the treatment of Phenylketonuria in our country, improving communication between family members and the care team, as well as identifying factors that help with treatment and adherence to the diet.

Please note that the interviews will be recorded and/or transcribed, that all information obtained will be considered confidential and that your identification will be kept confidential. The results of this study may be presented in scientific papers and events without any form of individual identification. Your participation is free and can be interrupted at any time.

If you agree to take part in this research by taking part in the Focus Group, the researcher asks you to sign this document in two copies.

Post-informed consent

Me ____

____
(Profession/function)

I declare that I have read and authorised my participation in the study "Diagnosis of Phenylketonuria: repercussions on the family and social relations". I also authorise the transcription of the interviews and their use for scientific research purposes.

I discussed my decision to take part in the research with the nutritionist in charge. The objectives and procedures to be carried out were clear to me

Legible signature

Contact telephone numbers: ____

____
Signature of the researcher responsible:

Rosângelis Del Lama Soares - CRN/MG: 0122CI   : M2-999880
Contact telephone numbers for the researcher: (31) 3285-1067 or (31) 99952-4789.

If you have any questions, you can contact the researcher, Rosângelis (Tel.: 3285-1067 / 9952-4789) or the UFMG Research Ethics Committee. Address: Av. Antônio Carlos, 6627. Administrative Unit II, 2° floor. Pampulha Campus. BH-MG. Brazil Tel: (31) 3409-4592.

Belo Horizonte, de de.

Analysing the data

The process of analysis is triggered by listening to the recorded material and starting the transcriptions. In qualitative clinical research, full transcriptions are usually the option, accurately reflecting the words of the interviewees and the interviewer. Thus, the speech of the various subjects should be transcribed in such a way as to recover the completeness of the statements (SIMIONI; LEFÈVRE; PEREIRA, 1996; TURATO; FONTANELLA; CAMPOS, 2006).

The data collected in the study was analysed using Content Analysis defined as:

> a set of communication analysis techniques aimed at obtaining, through systematic and objective procedures for describing the content of messages, indicators (quantitative or not) that allow the inference of knowledge related to the conditions of production/reception (inferred variables) of these messages (BARDIN, 2011, p. 37).

This technique was basically developed in four stages:

1) The pre-analysis took place on the basis of the transcribed material, gathering all the empirical material, reading it through, exhaustively exploring the content of each observation in the interviews and GF;

2) Once the material had been explored, coding was carried out, i.e. from the raw data the significant recording units were cut out by theme in order to reach the core of understanding of the text;

3) The data was then grouped by theme, making it possible to formulate the main categories;

4) Finally, the results were processed/analysed/studied, including inference and interpretation.

5) To describe and explain social phenomena, Content Analysis uses analytical categories that are constructed by breaking down the text into units (categories), identifying what they have in common, allowing them to be grouped together (CAREGNATO; MUTTI, 2006; POPE; MAYS, 2006).

According to Gomes (1999) and Minayo *et al.* (1994), a category is a concept that refers to elements with common characteristics or that are related to each other, enabling the researcher to establish classifications. Working with categories involves the procedure of grouping elements, ideas or expressions around a concept.

Triangulation is often used to maximise confidence in the validity of findings. It is a process that consists of looking at the object from different angles, comparing results between two or more data collection methods or sources of information, in which the researcher looks for patterns of convergence to develop or corroborate an overall interpretation (MINAYO, 2012; POPE; MAYS, 2006).

During the analysis process, the confrontation with literature data then has a complementary function, as a strategy for theoretical, methodological and data triangulation (DENZIM, 1970; MINAYO 2004; TURATO 2003; TURATO; FONTANELLA; CAMPOS, 2006).

Establishing links between findings obtained from different sources, illustrating them and making them more comprehensible can also lead to paradoxes, giving new directions to the problem under study (NEVES, 1993; TURATO; FONTANELLA; CAMPOS, 2006).

Minayo (2004, 2012) defends triangulation as an efficient form of validation and points to the importance of interaction between the researcher and the social actors, and the theoretical basis for evaluating the data, beyond what is being shown. She considers comparison to be a fundamental resource for guaranteeing greater universality of knowledge and, from a technical point of view, according to her, authors who work with qualitative research propose triangulation as an efficient proof of validation. For the author, good research usually involves comparing the data produced with other work that has already been carried out or, even better, started from it. She also reveals that a scientific attitude recognises the approximate nature of knowledge, i.e. the act of knowing is always unfinished, never complete. Therefore, the trustworthiness of the various points of view was sought in order to guarantee the diversity of meanings expressed by the interlocutors, thus avoiding the idea of a single truth.

Throughout the process of analysing the data in the two stages, triangulation was carried out with the researchers and the related literature.

The fact that the researcher was a member of the multi-professional team could have led to interpretation bias. To minimise this possible bias, the researcher had the help of her supervisor in analysing the transcribed material, as she is not a member of this team.

On the other hand, it is recommended that the researcher should be immersed in the context of the study, thus allowing for greater depth in understanding the reality being investigated. According to Minayo, 1994; Turato; Fontanella; Campos, 2006, the participation of the researcher as a mediating agent between the analysis and the production of information is considered positive during the research process. It is therefore important for there to be interaction between the researcher and the research subjects, since both parties are seeking mutual understanding.

At the end of the study, a methodological triangulation can be made between the different qualitative techniques used at each stage.

Quality in qualitative research

Good quality qualitative research must be relevant in some way to the population being studied. It hardly ends in itself: it is always open to discussion, to the possibility of adding new elements and the more debate it provides, the better its contribution to the scientific community will be (POPE; MAYS 2006).

Quality designates the essential part of things, what is most important and decisive, and signals the horizon of intensity, beyond extension. It signifies another dimension of qualitative phenomena that seeks depth and fulfilment. In short, it is a challenge of permanent rescue and persistent renewal (DEMO, 1998).

For Turato (2003), the greatest strength and relevance of qualitative studies, from the point of view of building knowledge, lies in their validity. The author sees internal validation as a process that involves the author and their project respecting standards that ensure truth based on the role of the researcher, the resources and instruments used in the research. The data is accepted as valid through the use of the set of knowledge and experiences that make up the researcher's intuitive, intellectual and technical base.

In this way, the author's professional background and the fact that she has been working with phenylketonuric patients and their families for more than sixteen years have allowed this study to safeguard the necessary precautions for its internal validity.

External validation, in clinical-qualitative research, would be:

> a process involving the author in possession of the research findings and their academic interlocutors, from whose interaction or intellectual affective debate would come favourable or adverse considerations to the attribute of truth of these findings (TURATO, 2003, p. 391).

Qualitative studies do not set out to generalise the results they produce. In this way, the validity of the study cannot be based on the possibility of generalisations. The validation of this research is based on diversity, on the reality laid bare, from the human complexity based on the singularity of the subjects investigated.

Ethical considerations

This study was considered feasible within the scope of the Centre for Action and Research in Diagnostic Support of the Faculty of Medicine of UFMG

(NUPAD-FM-UFMG) and approved by its Board of Directors. It was submitted to the Paediatrics Department of the Faculty of Medicine, the Paediatrics Functional Unit of the Hospital das Clínicas (HC), the Teaching, Research and Extension Directorate of the HC-UFMG and approved by the UFMG Research Ethics Committee (COEP-UFMG), process CAAE 0525.0.203.000-09 on 04/12/2009.

The mothers interviewed and the professionals from the multi-professional team were informed about the purposes of the study, objectives and methods explained in the Terms of Free and Informed Consent.
Informed Consent Form (ICF). The participation of all research subjects was conditional on reading and signing these documents, as shown in Figures 5.2 and 5.3.

The researchers undertook to keep the confidential data confidential and to guarantee the anonymity of the research participants in publications and presentations, ensuring their privacy.

The questions and doubts raised by the mothers before, during or immediately after the interviews were taken on board, clarified immediately after the interviews or referred for resolution and action. The results of the referrals were informed in due course to the mothers concerned.

The data obtained in this study will be used exclusively for scientific purposes, and access to it will be restricted to the researchers and members of the committee who took part in the Qualifying Exam and Thesis Defence. The recordings and transcripts of the interviews will remain in the author's custody for five years and will then be destroyed.

Results

> *"Every word always has a further meaning, it supports many functions, it involves many meanings. Behind what a discourse says, there is what it wants to say, and behind what it wants to say, there is yet another wanting to say, and nothing will ever be exhausted."*

The presentation of the results was organised into chapters six and seven, respectively. The sixth chapter presents mothers' perceptions of the repercussions of Phenylketonuria on family dynamics. Mothers of children aged two to six with an early diagnosis of Phenylketonuria, screened by the Minas Gerais State Neonatal Screening Programme and undergoing regular treatment at the Reference Service, were interviewed.

The seventh chapter discusses the perception of the multi-professional team about the care and treatment of the disease. For this investigation, a Focus Group was held with eight professionals from the Reference Service who treat phenylketonuric patients and their families.

CHAPTER 6

Maternal perception of the repercussions of phenylketonuria on family dynamics

Introduction

Phenylketonuria (PKU) is one of the most common metabolic disorders, transmitted genetically in an autosomal recessive manner. It is the most severe of the hyperphenylalaninemias (HPA) and is characterised by the absence or deficiency of the enzyme phenylalanine hydroxylase (PAH), synthesised by the liver, which is responsible for converting phenylalanine (phe) into tyrosine (tyr), leading to an accumulation of phe in the blood (CORNEJO; RAIMANN, 2010; MARTINS; FISBERG; SCHIMIDT, 1993; SCRIVER; KAUFMAN, 2001).

PKU is usually identified by neonatal screening carried out between the third and fifth day of the child's life. This condition allows for early treatment, preferably up to 21 days of age, which is essential for the normal growth and development of affected children. The most serious clinical manifestation of PKU is irreversible mental retardation (STARLING *et al.*, 1999).

The Minas Gerais State Neonatal Screening Programme (PETN-MG) was created in 1993 and is coordinated by the State Health Department. The Centre for Action and Research in Diagnostic Support of the Faculty of Medicine of the Federal University of Minas Gerais (NUPAD-FM-UFMG) is the programme's executing body, responsible for the treatment and laboratory tests carried out in the state's 853 municipalities to screen for Phenylketonuria, Congenital Hypothyroidism, Sickle Cell Anaemia, Cystic Fibrosis, Biotinidase Deficiency and Congenital Adrenal Hyperplasia.

The treatment of PKU is dietary and consists of a significant restriction of proteins. It should be started as soon as the diagnosis is suspected in order to avoid irreversible mental retardation. In order to adapt the diet to the protein needs of the affected individual, the Phe-restricted diet must be associated with a Phe-free or Phe-poor protein substitute. Individuals with PKU should maintain the diet for the rest of their lives, as its interruption is associated with a worsening of the Intellectual Quotient (IQ) in schoolchildren and a decrease in attention and speed of information processing in adults (NATIONAL INSTITUTES OF HEALTH, 2001).

Clinical and nutritional monitoring of PKU patients in the state of Minas Gerais is carried out by a multi-professional team and is centralised in Belo Horizonte, at the Phenylketonuria Outpatient Clinic of the Special Genetics Service of the Hospital das Clínicas of the Federal University of Minas Gerais (SEG-HC-UFMG). It is free, offered by the SUS, and guaranteed to all phenylketonuric patients living in Minas Gerais, whether or not they have been screened by the programme (KANUFRE *et. al*, 2001a).

The impact of PKU is often traumatic and disorganising for families. Regardless of the levels of stability at the time of diagnosis, many families need support to adjust to the new demands. From the moment of diagnosis, the family's activities become centred on the existence of this disease, ratified by the imperative use of a strict diet, different from that used culturally. Thus, in the day-to-day care of patients and their families, there is a complex experience that is not only explained by the disease itself. It often means radical changes in the lives of these people, who seek an alternative diet, different from the culturally established one, altering their family and social roles to some degree (SCHILD, 1972).

There are few studies in the literature that have dealt with living with the disease, its repercussions, and the emotional and psychological aspects involved in treating PKU.

Awiszus & Unger (1990), through interviews with parents, reported that the most important problem, from the families' point of view, was managing the diet, accompanied by experiences of loss and guilt.

The study by Russel, Mills and Zucconi (1988) found that shock and disbelief associated with fear and anxiety are reactions commonly reported by parents in relation to the diagnosis of PKU.

Considering that there are a large number of PKU patients in the Minas Gerais Reference Service (SR) compared to other countries, the importance of developing a study aimed at knowledge and understanding of the disease in family life is confirmed.

The aim of this study was to understand maternal perceptions of the repercussions of PKU on family dynamics and social circles, in the search for knowledge that could contribute to a more humanised and effective approach to treating the disease.

Method

This was a qualitative study. Mothers took part in the research, as they are privileged informants about the child's health and represent the majority of carers in the SR. Inclusion criteria were: being the mother of a child aged between two and six years old, with an early diagnosis of PKU and undergoing regular treatment at the Phenylketonuria Outpatient Clinic at SEG-HC-UFMG. Mothers with more than one child with PKU undergoing treatment were excluded, in order to study the disease situation as a new event in the family.

The mothers eligible for the study were identified by searching the NUPAD database, considering the period from 01/09/2010 to 31/03/2011. Forty mothers who met the inclusion criteria were found.

The semi-structured interview technique was used to collect data. Based on the review of related literature, the experience acquired by the researcher at the Phenylketonuria Outpatient Clinic and, in accordance with the objectives of the study, a six-question script was drawn up (Chart 6.1).

Table 6.1 **Interview questionnaire**

Questions
- What was it like to be told that your son had Phenylketonuria?
- What's it been like living with that?
- What has changed?
- How do you perceive your child's reaction to the diet?
- What are the biggest difficulties?
- How do you perceive the treatment and follow-up?

The mothers were recruited at the Centre for Education and Social Support (CEAPS), in the interval between the child's blood test for Phe and the appointment at the Phenylketonuria Outpatient Clinic at SEG-HC-UFMG.

After introducing the researcher, a brief explanation of the research was given and the Informed Consent Form (Figure 5.1) was signed. A questionnaire was then administered to characterise the mothers and their children with PKU (Figure 5.2), including clinical and sociodemographic information, with a view to identifying aspects that could contribute to understanding the reality under study.

All the interviews followed the established script and were recorded on MP3 with the informant's authorisation. The interviews lasted between 18 and 39 minutes. The anonymity of the participating mothers was guaranteed, and they were identified in their reports in the chronological order in which the interviews took place. All the interviews were transcribed by the researcher with the help of two undergraduate students from the Nutrition programme at the Federal University of Minas Gerais.

Fourteen mothers were interviewed and there were no refusals. The group of participants was closed when the information obtained in new interviews became repetitive and no longer contributed significantly to understanding the reality under investigation and to the theoretical reflection based on it. Thus, the saturation criterion was used to define the end of data collection

(FONTANELLA; RICAS; TURATO, 2008; MINAYO, 2004).

To analyse the material collected, we used the Content Analysis technique in the thematic modality (BARDIN, 2011). The main categories were then identified. The final analysis took place with the treatment and interpretation of the results obtained. This work was approved by the Research Ethics Committee of the Federal University of Minas Gerais (COEP-UFMG), process CAAE 0525.0.203.000-09.

Results and discussion

The mothers interviewed and their children with PKU

The socio-demographic profile of the fourteen mothers interviewed is shown in Table 6.1.

Table 6.1 Profile of the mothers of phenylketonuric children interviewed (n = 14)

Features		N	%
Age (years)	> 25 e < 30	8 4	57,2
	> 30 e < 35	1	28,6
	> 35 e < 45	1	7,1
	>45		7,1
Number of children	1	7	50,0
	2 or more	7	50,0
Lives with the child's father	Yes	13	92,9
	No	1	7,1
Consanguinity between parents	Yes	4	28,6
	No	10	71,4
Education	Illiterate	1	7,1
	Elementary incomplete	2	14,3
	Elementary complete High	4	28,6
	school incomplete	1	7,1
	Completed high school	3	21,5
	Superior	2	14,3
	Postgraduate studies	1	7,1
Family income in Minimum Wage (MW)	<1	1	7,1
	≥ 1 e<3	7	50,0
	≥3e<6	2	14,3
	≥6e< 10	2	14,3
	≥ 10	2	14,3
Works outside the home	Yes	7	50,0
	No	7	50,0
Religion	Seventh-day Adventist °	1	7,1
	Spiritist	2	14,3
	None	2	14,3
	Evangelical	4	28,6
	Catholic	5	35,7
Contacting the Basic Health Unit (UBS)	Yes	13	92,0
	No	1	7,1

	<50	6	42,9
Distance between municipality of origin and reference centre (Km)	≥50e< 120	1	7,1
	≥ 120 e< 250	4	28,6
	≥ 250 e < 400	1	7,1
	≥400	2	14,3
Difficulties with Treatment Away from Home (TFD) (*)	Yes	5	35,7
	No	6	42,9
	Not used	3	21,4
Receives financial aid	Yes	3	21,4
	No	11	78,6

Source: **NUPAD, 2013**[2]

(*) Benefit relating to transport, offered by local councils, for the treatment of patients in the SR, when it is located outside their municipality of origin.

The mothers were aged between twenty-five and forty-seven, with a median of thirty-six and a half (36.5) years. Only one did not live with the child's father.

Of the fourteen mothers interviewed, eleven (78.6 per cent) had at least completed primary school, three (21.4 per cent) had higher education and one (7.1 per cent) had a postgraduate degree.

Six (42.9%) of the mothers interviewed reported a family income of more than three minimum wages (MW). The Catholic religion was the most common, reported by five mothers (35.7%), followed by the Evangelical religion, with four mothers (28.6%) practising it.

Most of the mothers (13) maintained contact with the Basic Health Unit (UBS). Half of them lived more than 120 kilometres away from the SR, with the furthest residence being approximately 500 kilometres away. Some municipalities have difficulties making it possible for these families to come to the SR.

Treatment away from home (TFD) is a benefit offered by municipalities to families, guaranteed by a federal ordinance issued by the Secretariat of Health Care. It refers to the transport of patients to the SR, when this is not offered in the municipality itself. However, this benefit is not granted to

---

[2] DIAGNOSTIC SUPPORT RESEARCH CENTRE - NUPAD. Database.xlsx. [personal message]. Message received by <rodls@terra.com.br>. on 12 Nov. 2013.

families who live in places considered to be close to where the treatment takes place. Therefore, mothers who live in the metropolitan region of Belo Horizonte also have to come on their own, a situation that often poses a problem for families, especially the poorest ones.

The most common means of transport used to get to the ER are ambulances, vans or intercity buses. Five of the mothers interviewed (35.7%) complained that they have a lot of difficulty and are not always able to receive the benefit. Three families (21.5%) don't use the TFD. One of them because it was difficult for the municipality to release the benefit; the other because she didn't receive the benefit and the last because she lived far from where the transport departed.The majority of the mothers, 78.6%, (11) reported not receiving any financial support. Of the three (21.4%) who said they received aid, two were covered by the Bolsa Família programme and the third received a minimum wage as a benefit guaranteed to the child by court action.Table 6.2 shows the characteristics of the phenylketonuric children whose mothers were interviewed.

Table 6.2 **Profile of the phenylketonuric children whose mothers were interviewed (n = 14)**

Features		N	%
Sex		9	64,3
	Male Female	5	35,7
Age (years)		5	35,7
	>2e<3	3	21,5
	>3e<4 > 4 e < 5	1	7,1
	S5e<6	5	35,7
Age at first appointment (days)	> 15 e <22	7	50,0
	> 22 e < 29	5	35,7
	> 29 e < 34	2	14,3
Percentage of children attending appointments (%)	<70	1	7,1
	> 70 e < 80	3	21,5
	> 80 e < 90	3	21,5
	> 90 e < 100	5	35,7
	100	2	14,3
Type of hyperphenylalaninaemia	Classic PKU (*) Mild PKU (**)	7	50,0
		7	50,0
Report of an eating disorder	Yes No	4	28,6
		10	71,4
Adequate control by age group (average blood phe in pcromol/L)	No 1° year	14 11	100,0
	No 2° year	7	78,6
	No 3° year	5	50,0
	No 4° year	2	35,7

| | No 5° year | | 14,3 |

Source: **NUPAD, 2013.**[3]
(*) Blood phe reference value: > 1200 pmol/L (**) Blood phe reference value: 600 to 1200 pmol/L

Most of the children whose mothers were interviewed were male and their ages at their first appointment ranged from fifteen to thirty-four days, with an average of twenty-three (23) days and a median of twenty-four and a half (24.5) days. It's worth pointing out that half of the children (7) arrived for their first appointment at twenty-one (21) days old. Considering that the average time between receiving the blood sample, processing it and the laboratory releasing the result is less than two days (1.95 days), this is an adequate time between the screening test and the start of treatment. All the children underwent the overload test in the sixth month of life, in accordance with the SR care protocol.

Of the two children who arrived later for their first appointment (> 29 and < 34), one had a neonatal screening test carried out in a private laboratory on the ninth day of life (9°). The result took fifteen (15) days to be released and the family had difficulties finding the SR to start treatment. The other child's screening was carried out at twenty (20) days of age. The delay was further exacerbated by the fact that the family lived in an area that was difficult to access, in a town a long way from the state capital, and started treatment at thirty-four (34) days.

In this study, half of the children whose mothers were interviewed had an attendance rate of between 90 and 100 per cent, and two of them didn't miss any appointments.

With regard to adherence to the diet, ten of the mothers interviewed (71.4%) reported that their child did not break the diet and four of them (28.6%) said that dietary transgressions did occur. Of the children who did

---

[3] DIAGNOSTIC SUPPORT RESEARCH CENTRE - NUPAD. Database.xlsx. [personal message]. Message received by <rodls@terra.com.br>. on 12 Nov. 2013.

break their diet, only one was under the age of three.

With regard to blood levels of phe, there was greater control in the first year of life, when all the children had satisfactory results, within the reference values. From the second year onwards, this control has been declining, due to transgressions in quality or quantity, i.e. use of non-permitted foods or increased intake of permitted foods, respectively. It can be seen that by the third year of life, only half of the children whose mothers were interviewed (7) showed good biochemical control.

Analysing interviews with mothers

During the analysis of the transcribed material, the data was grouped by theme and, by means of a classification process, the main categories and their subdivisions were identified, as shown in Table 6.2.

Chart 6: Categories and subcategories identified in interviews with mothers

Categories	Sub-categories
A. Revealing the diagnosis	A.1 Maternal perception of the communication of a change in the neonatal screening test and referral to the Reference Service. A.2 Arriving at the first appointment at the Reference Centre
B. Learning to cope with illness	8.1 0 disease stigma 8.2 Maternal reactions to living with the disease 8.3 0 treatment 8.4 Strategies, suggestions and expectations
C. Implications of Phenylketonuria for the family and social circle	C.1 Economic implications for the family C.2 The child in the family and social environment C.3 Children at school

A. Revealing the diagnosis

A.1 Maternal perception of reporting a change in the neonatal screening test and referral to the Reference Service

Diagnosis in neonatal screening seems to invert the logic of the usual diagnosis in paediatrics. Generally, the parents of a child who is ill seek a diagnosis or guidance that explains their child's situation in order to resolve it. At the screening, the child is fine, without any sign of illness, giving the parents the pleasures of birth, when someone knocks on the door and informs them: 'This is not the newborn you're celebrating. He may have a problem and the problem may be serious'. And so, after this information, the celebration is interrupted by the shock of bad news.

According to Canguilhem (2006, p.58),

> Disease, which never existed in human consciousness, now exists in medical science. Doctors have clinical information and laboratory techniques that allow them to know that people who don't feel sick are sick.

For the author, there is no inversion of logic when it comes to identifying the diagnosis.

> The disease that can be prevented in advance by medical knowledge is logical, because it sends a message about the possibility of its appearance, avoiding serious and irreversible repercussions. He also points out that it takes lucidity and courage not to prefer an idea of illness, in which there may be some feeling of individual guilt, to an explanation of the illness with causality in the family genome. An inheritance that the heir cannot refuse, since inheritance and heir are one and the same (p. 240).

Despite being an almost unavoidable task for the doctor, breaking bad news to a patient or family member remains a difficult and special part of the health professional's job. The diagnosis of a serious illness, which involves the risk of death, disability and other losses, provokes intense and painful feelings. Bad news has been defined as any information that involves a drastic negative change in the affected individual's future prospects (PIRES, 1998).

So reporting a change in the neonatal screening test usually has a big impact, triggering immediate reactions of fright, shock, disorientation and anger.

> *"At first it was a huge scare because we always hope for a healthy child. [...]It's very scary."*

> *"I think it hit me at a time when I was very weak psychologically, you know? [...] Then the news came".*

The way in which the news of the suspected diagnosis of PKU is given can also accentuate the impact of the disease, with implications beyond the emotional aspects that can interfere and perpetuate throughout treatment. In addition to the fright, in several interviews the mothers also reported that they received the news of the disease without any preparation.

> *"The way she said it was like that, I don't know, all of a sudden, you know? [...] It scared the hell out of me, because at first glance, I honestly thought my son was dying."*

> *"The boy [...] came in saying the worst thing, that the baby had a very serious illness and would have been born with mental retardation. It interfered with breastfeeding, I couldn't feed the baby."*

There were also questions in some reports about the lack of knowledge of the disease among the health professionals involved in Newborn Screening.

> *"To me, what she told me was the same as nothing. She just came in and said that there was a change in his foot test, but not to worry, because at most he was going to have a different milk."*

> *"When I heard the news, I called his paediatrician, but she*

Regardless of professional training, as this is a rare disease, it is often observed that professionals do not have adequate knowledge about the illness; for this reason, they are unable to clarify or deal with the diagnosis and this can aggravate the shock and trigger panic.

Among the mothers interviewed, one of them revealed the path to her son's PKU diagnosis, starting with a sample taken from a private laboratory.

> *"I got him at the hospital. All private. After five days, he was tested and there was a slight change. [...] the paediatrician asked us to do it again. At the private laboratory again. We went to about four doctors and none of them knew. None of them said: 'Oh, you have to go to NUPAD for a reference'. No, none of the three paediatricians.*

In RS there is a well-established and successful flow in the public network (SUS) for the treatment of diseases identified by neonatal screening. All planning is geared towards minimising diagnosis time, and there is no similarity in the private service. As a result, erroneous referrals can lead to delays in diagnosis and the start of treatment.

When a child is identified as having a suspected diagnosis of PKU, a process is set in motion to speed up their arrival at the ER, which means that mothers and children have to travel immediately from their home town to Belo Horizonte.

The sudden approach made by the UBS professionals with a view to an urgent trip is revealed in the following statement:

> *"He came in and said: 'Hey, pack your bag because in half an hour you have to be travelling'. He had no skill.*

The lack of professional skills to make this referral urgently and the necessary agility to provide the first care and start treatment could alarm the family even more, causing destabilisation. On the other hand, if the appointment were delayed, the child would be subject to the repercussions of the delay in starting treatment, increasing the risk of neurological sequelae. In addition, the parents would probably be very worried and anxious about the unclear diagnosis, waiting for the first appointment.

It should also be noted that the state's vast territory means that many families of affected children have to travel long distances to the health centre. As described in Table 6.1, more than half of the mothers interviewed lived at least 50 km away from the health centre and two of them lived more than 400 km away from the health centre. This condition can also interfere with the organisation of municipalities to make it possible for these families to come to appointments and, consequently, to control and adhere to treatment. For this reason, it is necessary for professionals to be able to approach these families in a more prudent and appropriate manner.

A.2 Arriving at the first appointment at the Reference Centre

On the first day of treatment at the SR, the mother hopes that her child doesn't have the disease, which is when the denial phase kicks in.

> *"[...] we were very well-received, very well-welcomed. It was a day of great expectation, we were anxious because deep down we wanted the result to be the opposite of what we were expecting, right?"*

All newborns referred to the SR undergo a new phe blood test on the day of their first consultation at the Phenylketonuria Outpatient Clinic at SEG-HC-UFMG. After the geneticist's assessment and according to this new dosage, probable diagnoses are made and specific treatment is carried out.

> *"That's when the world came crashing down on me, what Phenylketonuria was."*

> *"When we got here and realised that we had to come every Wednesday, that distance, that diet, I was already worried about breast milk. If I could breastfeed [...]".*

When the results confirm the suspected diagnosis of PKU, at this point, despite the discouragement that the ratification of the diagnosis may bring, it's time to move on.

now, parents are better informed about the disease. They know that it is a chronic condition, that weekly appointments will begin and that the child will be treated for life. They are also informed that blood samples will be taken frequently, in addition to the daily use of a strict diet associated with a special formula that is essential for treatment. In short, a radical change in their lives, with the possibility of triggering a new impact. This time, the shock may be more evident with manifestations of great suffering, crying and anguish.

Awzius and Unger (1990) interviewed carers of phenylketonuric children about their experiences with treatment during the first year of life. The authors showed that the main problem faced at the time of birth was accepting the diagnosis. An experience described as a shock and lived with an extreme sense of guilt. They also noted feelings of denial, anger and difficulty believing that the treatment is for life.

B. Learning to cope with illness

2.1 The stigma of the disease

The presence of a chronic disease (CD) can be seen as a lifelong burden.

In the case of PKU, which is still little known, it carries the stigma of a disease marked by neurological sequelae and mental retardation.

For Goffman (1988), stigma reveals an individual's social identity and can be related to social class, ethnicity, profession or illness. A stigmatised individual is one whose real identity includes any attribute that frustrates expectations of normality. The author describes that a stigmatic illness can define someone as marked, undesirable or disadvantaged, which makes them feel ashamed, inferior or unacceptable in their environment.

Based on the assumption that people with CD have an attribute that makes them different from others, they can be or feel stigmatised, as the mothers interviewed revealed.

> *"When she told me she had a problem, I thought that was it: she wasn't going to walk, she wasn't going to talk, she wasn't going to listen."*

> *"I only saw that part of the information that was mental retardation, serious sequelae. Retardation for me is a very heavy word."*

The mothers also reported that some feelings persisted throughout the treatment. A fear related to the possibility of damage to the children's development, despite the early diagnosis. The fear of death, mental retardation and incapacity, generating fear and panic in families, above all because of the uncertain future and the difficulties of dealing with the illness throughout the child's life.

> *"Then, at the second consultation, when I saw the boys with problems, I started to feel bad, you know? So I thought, 'My God, is mine going to grow up to be like this?*

Thus, the stigma of PKU becomes yet another challenge in living with the disease, in the search for the social integration of these affected individuals, with a view to a healthy and appropriate family dynamic for all its members.

2.2 Maternal reactions to living with the disease

Following the news of the diagnosis, several maternal reactions are described, which can last for many years. In their testimonies, the mothers revealed their reactions to living with PKU and at the same time showed how they learnt to cope with the disease.

> *"A child with phenyl is not that big of a deal, but it is. It's a treatment that if you don't adapt to, you'll end up with sequelae. It's tiring, but it's worth it."*

Kubler-Ross (2000) describes the various stages that can be experienced by patients and their families in the face of serious illness. These include denial, anger, bargaining, depression, acceptance and hope. The author sees these as a healthy way of dealing with the painful and unpleasant situations that occur during the diagnosis and treatment of an illness, especially those of a chronic nature. Five of these six stages could be identified in the speeches of the mothers interviewed.

The first stage is characterised by a feeling of denial, which can act as protection so that the new situation can be assimilated.

> *"At first, even though I didn't say anything, I kept to myself. Sometimes I didn't even look. I'd read it and say: 'No, my son doesn't have that'. I didn't accept it".*

> *"I was very scared. I didn't want her (the child). I didn't want a sick child. I could give it to someone who didn't have a child. I didn't want to go near her.*

In the second stage, anger arises when denial can no longer be maintained. At this stage, feelings of loneliness, isolation and flight are common defence attitudes. For family and friends, this is a difficult phase to deal with.

> *"Why did this doctor come and say this to me, that it's for the rest of my life? Is he God? When I look at him, it makes me angry that he says it's for the rest of my life."*

Bargaining can be identified at a third stage, as an attempt at an advance, a promise, a prize, offered for good behaviour. It can be manifested by asking for a grace through an exchange. In this study, bargaining did not emerge clearly and objectively in the statements of the mothers interviewed.

The fourth stage is described as depression. The author emphasises the need for attention so that the symptom is not silenced and appropriate interventions can be carried out. Only people who manage to overcome their anguish and anxiety are able to find a different way of facing reality.

> *"I even went into depression. I wouldn't get up, I wouldn't eat, so I think I went a bit crazy in the head."*

The fifth stage describes acceptance of the illness. A phase of adaptation, where anger and envy will no longer be present towards those who will no longer be forced to submit to limitations in their daily lives.

> *"I think the important thing is to see him alive. Being able to live with your child. Today I realise that it's not something out of this world, right? There are worse things.*

Hope is the sixth stage and seems to persist throughout the different stages of life. Although lifelong treatment is recommended, some mothers expressed hope for a cure.

> *"[...] But we will never lose hope that God can heal the person from one moment to the next, at any moment."*

> *"She doesn't eat anything she can't. I trust her a lot. She sees cases here and says: 'Mum, if I eat, will I get this'? She asks God a lot to heal her and I tell her that nothing is impossible for God, right?*

In some of the testimonies, it was noted that hope combined with faith and religion can act as a structuring axis during treatment. As can be seen in Table 6.1, twelve of the mothers interviewed (85.7%) reported having a religion.

> *"As it is, we're going to ask God to help us take care of him, so that he stays healthy. He'll treat him well, won't he?"*

This last stage is marked by the need to understand the illness, going beyond the physical and biological limits. They look to God for answers to their questions, placing him as the driver of everything that happens in people's lives. They have to accept it, because they believe that He knows what He's doing (MOREIRA; DUPAS 2006).

Guilt is also a feeling that usually arises when PKU is diagnosed and can persist or recur throughout treatment, when related to dietary transgression in the face of the possibility of damage to children's development.

> *"I feel guilty when I get the results at the hospital. I think: Wow, I have to improve (the child's) diet because I'm afraid she'll have a problem. Then I worry about changing it, you know?*

In this study, resilience behaviours were also observed in the testimony of some of the mothers interviewed. Resilience is a concept that has been used to explain the ability that some individuals have to deal with problems, withstand adverse situations such as shock or stress, without going into psychological overdrive. The term refers to an ability to overcome adversity, which does not mean that the individual comes out of the crisis unscathed (ARAÚJO; MELLO; RIOS, 2011; YUNES, 2003).

> *"I got home, knelt at the foot of my bed and cried a lot. Then I said to God: 'I'm going to cry today as much as I have to, because I'm never going to cry again. As far as I'm concerned, she'll have a normal life. From that day on I got out of bed and went to look after her. And that's what I've been doing to this day.*

> *"Look, it was difficult at first, but as soon as he developed, we realised that it wasn't as horrible, as difficult as we thought."*

Damião and Ângelo (2001) reported that, over time, some families manage to realise that chronic illness (CD) is manageable, that it really is possible to live with it and think about a future for the child, by using coping strategies, accepting the illness and mastering the situation with more confidence and resourcefulness.

2.3 The treatment

Bearing in mind that clinical-nutritional follow-up is centralised in Belo Horizonte, one of the major difficulties encountered is the need for families to travel frequently throughout the course of treatment.Some mothers reported the difficulties they experienced when travelling to appointments.

> *"It's very difficult, especially because you have to expose a child, a little baby, to so many journeys, long distances, in a town hall car."*

> *"She (the child) gets very tired, you know. Her body hurts. On the way back she's more tired and gets a bit nauseous, cries [...]."*

Especially for families who live outside Belo Horizonte, travelling back and forth can be a huge sacrifice, especially in the first year of life. In the first six months alone, patients and their families travelled to the ER twenty times, and by the time they were a year old, they had travelled thirty-two times. In this study, only one of the mothers interviewed lived in Belo Horizonte.

Thus, the treatment recommended for life requires more from the family than just the availability of time. It requires dedication, the reorientation of finances, the reorganisation of tasks and all the commitment centred on one of its members, in an attempt to structure life based on this new circumstance.

In addition to the continuous travelling, one of the mothers reported the difficulty of leaving other children at home without assistance.

"When I come here, the girls stay there on their own, one goes to school and the other comes and watches her (24-year-old disabled daughter with a late diagnosis of PKU without treatment at the family's option). I worry about them there. I get worried, but you have to treat it, right? You can't leave him untreated.

In this way, the treatment causes the mother to distance herself from the home and other members of the family. This distancing also can alter family relationships, further jeopardising coping with the situation.

Another issue highlighted by the mothers was the difficulty with Out-of-Home Treatment (OHT). Despite being a regulated benefit, the flow is not always satisfactory. Among the complaints reported are: lack of resources by the municipalities; lack of drivers; lack of vehicles, especially during election campaigns; vehicles in a poor state of repair and maintenance, creating insecurity for passengers; failure to release funds to families for alternative travel, such as their own cars or intercity buses.

Some mothers also complained that they come in ambulances, travelling for many hours with too many passengers, many patients in more serious medical conditions and with various pathologies.

The mothers also revealed their concerns about the journey home, as they are often pressurised by ambulance drivers to be released quickly from outpatient appointments.

One of the participating mothers also mentioned her wish to be accompanied by another family member, in addition to the child undergoing treatment, and that it wasn't possible.

Some children need to come with more than one companion, especially at the beginning of treatment, when the mother is more fragile and insecure. It's an opportunity for the father to be able to accompany her, including to learn more about the disease and treatment. There are still cases of patients with severe neurological and motor sequelae. However, it is difficult for the municipality to provide another seat on the transport offered.

Two of the mothers interviewed lived in rural areas and one of them said she had difficulty getting from rural to urban areas on the day of her son's appointment in Belo Horizonte.

> *"Those first few days I suffered so much that I even travelled on horseback to get to the city. My husband was taking me the little boy with his bag on his horse and I was walking. The mud and clay bogged down my legs. There were days when I wanted to turn back, but I had to go. It was all wet and I had to face it anyway. Then I said I couldn't stand it. Then they picked it up. They'll manage now. "*

Families living in rural areas are often far from the municipality and from the place where transport to Belo Horizonte leaves. To reach it, they have to walk for hours, or even ride a horse or cart in the early hours of the morning or late at night.

One of the mothers also reported that in her town there is no daily transport to the SR, so they stay in Belo Horizonte for more than two days. They sleep in shelters provided by the municipality of origin, and may return the next day or stay even longer.

> *"They pick you up at home two days before. I left home on Monday and didn't arrive until Thursday. Some days it's been a week, some days I cried wanting to leave when I didn't have a car."*

> *'I didn't even leave, did I? I used to stay at the house (a support centre in the municipality of origin). It was hard to find a place to go and come back. I'd stay for a couple of weeks or a month.*

From the start of neonatal screening in September 1993 until On 31 December 2012, 20,906 appointments were scheduled. These appointments resulted in an 83.4 per cent attendance rate, with 17,433 appointments, and for the age group in this study (two to six incomplete years) there were

approximately 87 per cent turnout (NUPAD, 2012)[4] .

As can be seen in Table 6.2, similar results were found in this study. Ten of the children whose mothers were interviewed attended at least 80 per cent of their scheduled appointments, and seven of them attended at least 90 per cent. The absences that led to missed appointments were for a variety of reasons, including maternal depression.

> *"Sometimes I miss appointments because of my depression. [...] Because some days I want to talk to God and everything, but some days I don't want to go out, I don't want to see anyone. So that affects me a lot.*

The percentage of absences from scheduled appointments is one of the indicators used to assess adherence to treatment (Table 6.2). For this reason, in recent years the Treatment Control Sector (SCT- NUPAD) has been improving this monitoring to check the reason for each absence, contacting the municipality of origin of the patient undergoing treatment.

Because it is a serious and rare disease, many mothers revealed in their testimonies that it is common to observe a lack of knowledge among doctors in the affected child's municipality of origin.

> *"I take him to the doctors there and I think they're very unprepared - they're scared. And phenylketonuria is not something to be afraid of."*

> *"Even when he was ill, the paediatricians didn't want to give him medicine because they didn't know if he could take it. I even had to call the doctor here to get a vaccine for him. The one made*

---

4 DIAGNOSTIC SUPPORT RESEARCH CENTRE - NUPAD. Database.xlsx. [personal message]. Message received by <rodls@terra.com.br>. on 12 Oct. 2012.

Parents and health professionals from different municipalities often contact the SR to clarify their doubts about diet, clinical symptoms, prescribing medication, administering vaccinations, etc.

The difficulty professionals have in providing care and managing the disease, coupled with the fact that treatment is totally centralised in Belo Horizonte, is one of the factors that can contribute to weakening the family's bond with the public health network in their municipality. It should also be emphasised that the fragmentation of care makes it difficult to monitor treatment, as well as contributing to the mythification of the disease.

From the age of two, visits to the SR are every two months, requiring a monthly blood sample to be taken in the municipality. In this regard, one of the mothers said she had difficulty getting this collection done.

> *"The last few times we've had the hardest time collecting. There, for example, the collection doesn't take place at the Health Centre in our region, you have to go elsewhere to collect it. And at great expense, because it's only one person who does it."*

Monthly blood sampling has been adopted by the SR protocol for over 15 years and is reinforced in all the monthly training sessions offered by NUPAD-FM-UFMG in Belo Horizonte to health professionals from all the municipalities in the state. Despite this, there are difficulties in carrying it out in several municipalities, one of the main allegations being the lack of professionals trained to carry out venous collection in children.

At CEAPS and the Phenylketonuria Outpatient Clinic, the bond between the mothers of children with early and late diagnoses comes naturally and is gradually consolidated by their shared condition and the solidarity between them.

If, on the one hand, SR-centred care is difficult, on the other, seeing other children diagnosed, treated and with good clinical progress makes mothers realise that treatment is possible, successful and prevents mental retardation.

> *"It's good for those of us who are just arriving. You have more courage, more strength. I don't want my son to be like that, because theirs was late."*

> *"Even if she starts treatment young, if I let her eat meat, beans, all those things she can't, the PKU she takes won't work. The test will only get bigger, and by the time I see it, everything inside her has burst."*

However, one of the mothers said she preferred not to have this meeting because she was intimidated by the situation.

> *"I keep thinking about my son looking like that, it bothers me. I'd rather not see it, it hurts our hearts. It pains me".*

Most of the children seen at the clinic are accompanied only by their mothers, as is the case with most children in Brazilian society. In the case of PKU, the father is asked at least once at the first appointment for genetic counselling and clarification of the diagnosis and treatment. At subsequent appointments, few fathers accompany mothers and their children with PKU. In this study, of the fourteen mothers interviewed, only two were regularly accompanied by their partners. Three of the mothers interviewed expressed how they felt.

> *"No, he never came, from the beginning it was just me and him. I'm left with a hole".*

> *"I've only been alone so far. He was here last year, just once. I'm the only one who heard everything.*

This routine, which is mainly the mother's responsibility, favours the onset of maternal loneliness. In general, the mother is almost exclusively responsible for caring for the child, while the father works to maintain the household. Nóbrega *et al.* (2012) also found this overload of tasks when they interviewed female carers. These women considered themselves to be the sole providers of childcare in different settings: family, home, hospital and community. It can be seen that
he gender issue is intrinsic to society, exerting strong cultural influences on the way mothers organise their lives and family routines in the face of the demands triggered by CD.

Gutierrez and Minayo (2010) also reported that when discussing health care within the family, the figure of the woman-mother as the main carer appears almost as a consensus, which means that care is almost synonymous with women. The woman-caregiver relationship is taken for granted because it is something that belongs to the domestic sphere. In this sense, we recommend investigating the conditions linked to the family structure in society and in the culture in which care must be produced.

In a study on PKU in the family, Brazier and Rowlands (2006) reported on the importance of improving these families' feelings of helplessness, dependence and isolation. The authors also revealed a mother's statement about the disease and treatment: *"Living with PKU will never be easy, but you have no choice but to move on and then live your life"* (p. 488).

It is the mother who has the opportunity to get to know patients with a late diagnosis and, as a result, reflect on and often imagine her own child in that condition. This anguish can bring ambiguous feelings of relief, fear and tension, as well as reinforcing the need for appropriate treatment.

> *"Then when he said something like: 'Oh my child, I could be giving you meat, but I can't. It makes me sad. It makes me sad'. I'd say: 'No, you're not, you've never seen the children who have*

problems there. Oh, you don't go to the consultation, so you don't have the right to say much here. I'm the only one who has to say anything. I even let him go out with her. I don't think he's daft enough to give it to her, because it shows on the test".

The mothers also said that the difficult management of the diet brings an overload of responsibilities and constant stress for them.

"His father, he's the kind of person who can't say no. So I have this spirit of leadership in my house, and it's not an advantage, because we get so overwhelmed. You're the only one who says no, you're the only one who makes decisions, you're the only one who calculates, you're the only one who measures. Only you impose the rules. So I got to a point where I really lost it.

In this study, many statements revealed that diet can become a source of conflict between the parents of a child with PKU. The maternal figure appears to have the greatest responsibility for the child and their treatment, and can feel very controlling and demanding.

"His father feels very sorry for him. He thinks that because he has Phenylketonuria, he doesn't have to charge for the rest. He thinks he can eat potatoes every day. Poor chap! He says: 'He can't eat this, he can't eat that, let him eat potatoes today'. I say: I won't let him [...] and that's that. That's it, understand? I swear. There have to be limits. Then they both get angry with me. His father says I'm the family's executioner. So we argue all the time.

"Dad is much more anxious, he finds it much harder to deal with the situation. At home I'm more centred and he's more permissive. He has a hard time dealing with no. When I say to him: She can't eat that. I can see that he feels like he's the child".

Parents seem to find it more difficult to control their child's diet. Sometimes, they become vulnerable to the behaviour of the affected child and, as a result, may allow certain dietary transgressions. When they are unable to impose themselves on the child, there can be scenes of antics, manipulation and a lack of boundaries.

On the other hand, it is common for mothers to take responsibility for caring for their children, especially when they require special attention. In the study by Awzius and Unger (1990), the children's fathers were only mentioned twice when talking about the diet, and one of the mothers said that when her husband realised that she could manage the diet on her own, he simply left the responsibility to her.

The importance of neonatal screening in enabling early diagnosis, appropriate treatment and a normal life for affected children was also mentioned.

> *"I'm grateful every day for the treatment I get, because I didn't have it before. Just looking at my daughter and seeing that she's normal gives me satisfaction. Every time I come here I see so many children who are becoming adults, all normal... It's an enormous source of happiness for me.*

It's interesting to note that although the Newborn Screening Programme is well known and publicised, the heel prick test is still met with resistance. One of the mothers interviewed revealed the conflict she had experienced with the PKU child's grandmother, who considered the test to be unnecessary suffering.

> *"We say: 'Blessed Little Foot Test'. Because it avoids a lot of suffering. Having the opportunity to get your child out of that situation is something else. It's one thing for a child to be born that way, but it's another thing to be able to give them the best. Then my mum always says: 'Imagine if you'd listened to me'. It's a good thing I'm big-headed.*

The mothers interviewed also revealed their opinions about treatment at the SR.

> *"For me, the treatment, the welcome here, there's nothing to complain about. It's the support you're giving us, so that our child*

grows up healthy."

"For me it's great, because you arrive, you have a support centre, you have doctors to clarify, to help you. I think that's very important".

Despite being satisfied with the reception and treatment, the mothers interviewed said they were tired and had to wait for their appointments, especially at the Phenylketonuria Outpatient Clinic at SEG-HC-UFMG.

"Here (at CEAPS) we chat, watch TV, have lunch, the kids play and we keep up with them, catch up, right? It's only when we get downstairs (to the clinic) that we're really tired! The day could go quickly so we could leave.

"The problem is the outpatient clinic, the space is very small, and we spend a lot of time there because there are so many children. They can't behave well, they shout, sometimes it even disturbs the consultation."

Considering the incidence of PKU in the state, it is expected that at least twelve new cases will be identified each year by the Minas Gerais Neonatal Screening Programme. This means that there is a progressive increase in the number of patients to be cared for, since the new cases are added to the old ones that will remain in treatment for life. As a result, new demands arise, such as frequent requests for reports, reports, referrals for specialised consultations, extending the time it takes to provide care and increasing the waiting time for patients to be released for each consultation.

One of the mothers interviewed made suggestions for filling this time.

"I think there could be a painting class, right? For mums, because the children already have one. Handicrafts would be good, a talk about phenyl, right?

Developing art-related projects in waiting rooms by multi-professional health teams could be used as a strategy to teach patients how to deal with their own health and to raise awareness of issues related to this topic (NAZARETH; SOUZA; FIGUEIREDO, 2007).

The mainstay of PKU treatment is a diet based on significant protein restriction combined with a protein substitute. The protein substitute, which is essential for treatment, is offered free of charge by the Unified Health System (SUS). In general, it is a formula based on free amino acids, free of or low in Phe, enriched with vitamins, minerals, selenium and tyr.

The main aim of treatment is to control dietary intake of Phe, keeping blood levels within the reference limits recommended for phenylketonurics in each age group. At the same time, it must provide an adequate supply of macro and micronutrients that allow the individual's growth and development to be maintained throughout life.

In the diet, the foods not allowed are all those of animal origin, pulses, wheat derivatives and diet products containing aspartame. Other foods such as rice, potatoes, vegetables, popcorn, juices and fruit in general are allowed in controlled quantities. Only foods and products based on vegetable oils and sugars are allowed, as well as honey (from the age of one), artificial powdered juices, soft drinks, cotton candy, candies and lollipops without milk. The diet should be individualised according to the tolerance levels observed over time and maintained throughout life (KANUFRE *et aL,* 2001a).

Powdered milk formulated for children up to six months of age has a lower concentration of Phe and is prescribed as part of the diet, whether or not it is combined with breast milk (STARLING, 2005). Unlike the protein substitute, its distribution is not guaranteed by the SUS and it is the family's responsibility to purchase it, which is often difficult due to the high cost. Even though it is not compulsory for the municipalities where the affected child comes from to offer it, some are sensitive to this demand, especially in the case of poorer families, and release it on prescription from a doctor or nutritionist.

One of the mothers interviewed reported her difficulty and discomfort in acquiring modified infant formula. In her view, she was entitled to receive it free of charge.

> *"When it comes to (the name of the infant milk formula), it's the hardest thing for them to supply. Because all the mums here get it. He's the only one who doesn't."*

From the start of treatment, in the first few days of life, the amino acid formula, free of phe, is offered in a bottle with good acceptance.

> *"The first year, the first moment, the impact I had was: Is this girl going to take this bottle? Then, from the moment she took it, she loved it, she suckled. Then I felt calmer.*

The majority of mothers revealed that it is very difficult to maintain an adequate intake of this protein substitute when replacing the bottle with a sippy cup.

> *"I've already noticed that without the bottle, he doesn't want to take the PKU otherwise. He won't take it. Then he thinks, he vomits."*

> *"I've tried putting it in a bottle, in those little cups. I've tried fruit and he won't take it either. The only way is in a bottle [...]".*

Considering the importance of drinking the special formula for PKU, there is a tolerance and even relaxation towards replacing the bottle with the cup from the age of two. For the children, there seems to be a conditioning of the taste of this special formula to the use of the bottle, making it difficult to accept it in other containers. There are children who still use the bottle at an advanced school age, making it difficult to remove it, which in turn can harm the child's emotional development, as well as their teeth.

One mum reported that her five-year-old son still uses a bottle and sucks on it until he falls asleep.

> *"I don't let him go to family parties, because he always does the wrong thing. The others go and he stays. Until he wants to go. I turn on the telly and give him toys. He watches woodpeckers and then takes a bottle of PKU and goes to sleep. He keeps the bottle in his mouth until it's dry.*

She uses this resource to calm him down whenever she needs to divert his attention away from food he can't eat. Or to distract him while his siblings go out partying, thus preventing him from breaking his diet.

The mothers interviewed revealed that, at the beginning of treatment, the diet is easier to manage and monitor.

> *"The first year was quiet, because he didn't demand anything, he was a child, a baby and he didn't have any will of his own, he didn't ask. So it was quiet."*
> *The child has less autonomy, she accepts what you give her, she doesn't ask for it. They want something different.*

> *"At first the child accepts everything, right? So, like, he accepted the PKU really well. So at first it's very good, but then, right? He says he's going to run away to buy sweets. So it's complicated."*

In the first few months of life, the child is completely dependent on the carer and when they adapt to the special amino acid formula, there are practically no difficulties in adhering to the treatment. Awzius and Unger (1990) also reported in their study that ten of the eleven carers interviewed said that the child had no problems accepting the diet throughout the first year of life.

The special amino acid formula has a peculiar flavour, characteristic of free amino acids, which is unpalatable and especially repulsive to non-phenylketonuric individuals. Di Ciommo *et. al.* (2012) mentioned that having PKU is difficult, not only because of the strict dietary restriction that must be maintained throughout life, but also because of the unpalatable special formula.

However, many children accept it very well, demanding more and treating it in a special way, as if it were chocolate milk.

"He can't do without this porridge. He asks for PKU, he says it's good. He eats it straight. That's the best thing that's happened. If he sees the tin, which is in the fridge
he says: 'Give me a little PKU. What a treat, what a treat'".

Although rare, the adverse effects of using this special formula can arise, as one of the mothers interviewed told us.

"He'd just taken the PKU, it wouldn't be 10 minutes and he'd have that black poo, that foam, that stench, that bad odour. And I always insisted: I think it's the PKU. And that conclusion was only reached after six months of suffering. He started to become malnourished and dehydrated. Then... (crying). But since it's the doctors' job and they were investigating hygiene issues, they had to understand everything. He had to undergo various tests, including faeces tests. Then, towards the end, after he was hospitalised here in the emergency room, you decided to take him off PKU for a week. After eight months he stopped pooing. He started to poo hard.

For infants, phe-free amino acid formula is combined with corn starch, sugar and sometimes vegetable oil. For this reason, it results in a product with a higher osmolarity than modified infant formulas (around 300 mOsm/kg of water), which can lead to gastrointestinal complications. Therefore, individual tolerance must always be taken into account.

The intake of the special formula for PKU should be divided into three to four portions a day, throughout the day and preferably after meals. Especially from school age onwards, adequate intake of this protein substitute can become a major difficulty at home, at school and in the social environment. This ideal consumption practice can also interfere with the affected individual's day-to-day activities, including their diet.

and often omit the existence of the disease out of embarrassment. Frank, Fitzgerald and Legge (2007), when investigating the social impact of restrictive diets for phenylketonurics and living with the disease, concluded that patients not only feel embarrassed and different from others because they can't eat what others eat around them, but also because they have to consume amino acid formula, something unfamiliar to the general population.

Two of the informants reported the difficulty of accepting and making feasible such a restrictive diet in relation to common everyday foods.

> *"Because as far as I was concerned, until I learnt about the disease, a person couldn't survive without meat, milk, eggs, beans, wheat flour or other things. All this is very important to me."*

> *"Look, the only thing that affects and changes a lot is food. Because we end up having to adapt the type of food he eats. All our lives we've eaten what we've always been used to eating and then, suddenly, it's time to change. It's complicated.*

The characteristics of the PKU diet are striking, both in terms of the limitation of foods and the non-use of those that have always been recognised as indispensable to life and the proper development of the individual. As a result, at the beginning of treatment, families experience a daily conflict, trying to adapt to the new situation.

One of the mothers also reported the difficulty she had in varying her child's diet.

> *"Look, for him to eat I have to put the rice in. He eats more rice,
> because there are times when there's nothing else. I have other
> things to eat, but he can't eat them. So I give him more rice.*

Low consumption of plant sources can be due to a lack of financial resources, the absence of this eating habit in the family, or the scarcity of these foods in certain municipalities. These are some of the situations that further aggravate the diversification of the diet which, in addition to being monotonous, can become very poor in nutrients.

When selecting processed foods, labels should also be checked for the protein content of the food per portion. In this respect, one of the mothers revealed a difficulty.

> *"[...] there are things we can't read and there are things I can't
> offer, because the nutritional table is only on the box. The
> caramel had nothing, no information, so I asked the girl and she
> said: 'Oh, it's because it comes in the box and I don't have the
> box anymore'. So, I think the nutritional table on the food leaves
> a lot to be desired. And there are some that don't even include
> protein [...]".*

Products packaged in multi-unit boxes are marketed at the retail level in individual portions and often do not contain a description of the nutrient composition on the original packaging label; since it is not possible to assess the composition of these foods, the phe content cannot be quantified and therefore safe consumption cannot be guaranteed.

Families are instructed on how to read and interpret the amount of protein in industrialised products per portion. This information is useful for quantifying the daily intake of phe from the food consumed. However, many mothers, regardless of their level of education, reported having difficulty calculating or feeling insecure about making the choice, as reported by one of the mothers with higher education.

According to Bekhof et. al (2003), low adherence to treatment is often a problem. The hypothesis that increased knowledge about the disease could improve diet control was not confirmed in the authors' study. They concluded that adherence to treatment is influenced by psychological and emotional aspects, and not just by knowledge of the disease.

This study corroborates the findings in the literature in that it identifies the importance of the psychosocial aspects involved in treatment, making it possible to devise strategies to deal with the disease and improve adherence to treatment, making it more effective.

There are few special products for PKU in Brazil and they are expensive compared to similar ones. However, there are patients who generally receive donations from some municipalities. One of the mothers reported her expectations regarding the acquisition of these special foods.

In general, industrialised products with a low Phe content are more expensive than similar products; they are bought by families or acquired by municipalities to donate to phenylketonurics. The Association of Parents and Friends of Phenylketonurics (APAFE) meets this demand by preparing special food baskets for PKU, containing a variety of handmade or industrialised products.

Awzius and Unger (1990) reported that the main challenges encountered were planning the menu, calculating the appropriate quantities of food, the cost of the diet and the doubt about having another child. The authors also revealed similar difficulties concerning: teaching the child about the nature of their illness; maintaining control of the child's diet throughout the day; making substitute foods available on special occasions; maintaining decisions about the child's diet. The study also concluded that, despite great concern about maintaining dietary goals and recognising the potential risks to the child's development, the majority of caregivers did not maintain an adequate diet.

Thus, the difficulty of accessing special foods makes the diet even more monotonous and unattractive, compromising the adequate intake of nutrients, a factor that favours dietary transgression. The scarcity of options means that mums have to prepare special recipes for PKU. However, some reported difficulties.

> "The *only difficulty is that we have to make the food at home, because we can't find it to buy. Most things we have to make ourselves."*

> *"I struggle in the kitchen, I'm still not great in the kitchen. I do, but it's difficult. Sometimes we work and don't have as much time to spend in the kitchen [...]".*

Preparing special recipes for PKU can be compromised by a lack of time to devote to cooking, a lack of financial resources to buy specific ingredients and a lack of cooking skills. In addition, as one of the mothers reported, even when resources are available, it is difficult to find quality foods with a low concentration of Phe that are suitable for consumption.

> *"When I go out shopping for my other child I take everything I can, that fits into my budget. For her (the child with PKU), even though I can afford to buy, I find very few things [...]. Very few*

Nalin *et al.* (2010) identified some difficulties in correctly adhering to dietary treatment for PKU, such as: limited information on the content of Phe in commercialised foods, a very restrictive diet that favoured a monotonous menu and difficulty in accessing products with a low protein content.

Archer et al. (1988) reported a case in which the family and the child treated early and continuously faced serious difficulties during mealtimes. The child's feeding problems began at a very early age, around one month old, and continued throughout the pre-school and school years. However, over time, the child showed adequate growth and development rates, and no behavioural problems, other than those related to eating, were diagnosed. These problems included being slow to eat a small amount of food, not accepting permitted foods and refusing to try new ones, as well as not eating the special formula. The child also had constant vomiting between the ages of three and six. He described eating as repulsive and said he felt excluded because he couldn't eat what other people ate. These difficulties were addressed when the parents and the child underwent therapeutic sessions and training in techniques to manage her eating behaviour. After six months of intervention, they reported facing fewer difficulties during family meals. In this family, the belief in the seriousness of the illness and the benefits of treatment favoured satisfactory engagement on the part of the parents, achieved above all by the balanced family environment.

Moreira and Dupas (2006) reported in their study that food restriction becomes much more difficult when the child is interacting with people who don't share this situation.

In this study, some mothers reported that as the years go by, children start to choose what they want to eat and compare their diet with that of others.

It is known that as children grow up, difficulties arise. Especially after the second year of life, when they begin to socialise with other members of their family and social circle. According to Table 6.2, in the first year of life, all fourteen children whose mothers were interviewed showed adequate control of their blood levels of phe. From the second year onwards, three of these children did not maintain control. Among the children who violated the diet, only one was under three years old, the others were between four and five years old. These findings corroborate those obtained in the SR, since adherence to the diet is practically complete in the first and second years of life. After this age, there is a tendency for adherence to decrease. Castro *et al.* (2012) in a study of 63 phenylketonuric patients between the ages of six and twelve in the state of Minas Gerais, observed that up to the age of two, 32 children (55%) showed better control of the average concentrations of phe in the blood. However, between two and six years of age, only 13 (20.6%) were considered to have good control. The authors also concluded that the results can be explained by the child's lesser autonomy up to the age of two, associated with the family's greater control over the activities carried out by the patients in the first years of life and, consequently, greater rigour in monitoring food intake.

Papalia and Olds (2000) also reported that until the second year of life, the family is usually the child's only reference point, making it easier to control their diet. At this stage, the child still experiences little and doesn't usually leave their parents or carers.

Children diagnosed with PKU at an early stage and undergoing regular treatment show no signs of the disease, since clinical manifestations appear between three and six months of age in untreated patients. This absence of signs, which in principle could be an advantage for affected children, can also lead to doubts about the existence of the disease, making it difficult to believe in the diagnosis and consequently the implication for treatment and adherence to the diet.

> *"... the sequelae, the retardation. I looked at him and there was no sign, no information".*

> *"I spoke to the school, I spoke to the counsellor, I made it very clear, I'm really scared, because it's a very serious thing. Sometimes they look and say: 'That boy has nothing'. The person doesn't believe it, they say that the mother is a shrew".*

> *"I usually leave (the child's name) with his (the husband's) family. But I'm really scared, you know? They say: 'She can eat, because she has nothing. That's rubbish, the girl is clever, you can give her to them. It won't hurt, just a little piece'".*

According to the SR protocol, all the children whose mothers were interviewed underwent an overload test in the sixth month of life to confirm the diagnosis. One of the mothers revealed that she had asked God for a cure.

> *"Yes, when he was six months old he had the test and we waited for it not to come back. I waited for the result, that it wouldn't work, that I wouldn't have the disease. That God was going to take that away... One more hope, right?*

Despite all the evidence pointing to the fact that the amount of phe ingested in the diet has a direct influence on the results of the blood tests, it has been observed during consultations at the Phenylketonuria Outpatient Clinic that many parents maintain the hope that the diagnosis will be reversed at this stage. This can be a time to relive the feelings of shock and disappointment triggered at the start of treatment.

However, one of the mothers reported that, after the overload test, she came to accept the diagnosis and treatment better.

> *"In the overload test, the test went up again. Then I think we accepted it more. I was already accepting it, because we already knew that the child would be normal, there would be nothing, no sequelae. It was just a matter of continuing the treatment.*

With the definition of the type of hyperphenylalaninaemia (HPA), families who were still reluctant to accept the disease may become more resigned to improving adherence to treatment, as well as acceptance.

When parents don't accept the diagnosis, and the denial phase is prolonged, the risk of dietary transgression increases, as one mother reported.

> *"Look, when he was younger, his father gave him a piece of sausage to try. And when he tastes it, he can smell it."*

Other reports indicate that good adherence to treatment is an attitude that starts with the family. Some children eat their meals at the table with the rest of the family, without the different menu causing any embarrassment. It's likely that this process has been built up since the beginning of treatment.

> *"He eats the little things I make for him. I've made pasties, cassava drumsticks. Every now and then I invent. [...] You can leave meat; fry an egg and leave it there and he (the child) won't touch it. He can barbecue and if someone from outside says: Here. He says: "I can't eat tutu (the meat is tutu)". So that means he's already getting to know what he can and can't eat." (1: child aged 3 years and 8 months)*
> *"I eat in front of him. He says 'meat smells bad Mum'.*

Therefore, there is evidence that when the family, from the beginning of the diagnosis, tries to impose a routine that favours treatment, the child may have less difficulty adhering to the diet.

In some of the testimonies, the mothers reported that the PKU diet changed the family's eating habits, with the inclusion or increase of plant sources and this change improved the quality of everyone's diet. In this sense, the disease brings the opportunity to change lifestyle habits, benefiting the whole family.

It should be emphasised that mealtimes can be a time for family education. However, although it is not recommended, it has also been observed that families try to deprive themselves of foods that are forbidden to phenylketonurics or, when they do consume them, they do so away from the child's eyes, on the sly, due to the difficulty of reconciling the family's diet with the diet offered to the child with PKU.

Family support for adherence to the diet is fundamental for proper control of the treatment, as one of the mothers interviewed reported.

According to Ferreira *etal.* (2012), the meanings of chronic illnesses do not belong exclusively to the sick individual. They are also the property of family members and the social network who, shared directly or indirectly, end up influencing the treatment and course of the illness.

Fiese and Everhart (2006) suggest that care management strategies for children with CD and a cohesive family climate can promote adherence to treatment over time. They reported that conflictual and disengaged family interactions tend to disrupt adherence and inevitably cause a decline in the child's health.

Alaei *et al.* (2011) in their study on the social status of the family and dietary adherence of PKU patients in the Iranian population reported that there was a significant association between divorced and unemployed parents with high levels of phe in the blood.

2.4 Strategies, suggestions and expectations

Throughout the course of treatment, as difficulties of all kinds are experienced, some strategies are identified and shared with other families. Among the main motivations is always the quest to improve adherence to the diet and the children's commitment to the treatment.

Some mothers reported strategies adopted to control the feeding of their child with PKU.

The internet was one of the most common ways of researching the disease and special foods for PKU. This type of strategy can be very useful not only for researching topics of interest, but also for exchanging ideas and clarifications with the SR, as one of the mothers interviewed reported.

"Often I have difficulty with something, I email here, I ask the (nutritionist) for help, [...]. We need this contact, and only you nutritionists can guide us."

Many families see the importance of talking to their children with PKU from an early age about treatment and dietary restrictions. There are those who, from the outset, don't change their routines at home, keeping the same food on the table, sharing meals and taking part in social gatherings. Ongoing awareness and education about diet control becomes a daily goal to be pursued. Four of the mothers interviewed reported how they deal with the disease.

"Ever since he was little, since he was on my lap I think, I always talked to him. People thought it was unnecessary for me to talk to him about it [...], he was so small. But today I see that it was very important. I trust him. He already talks to the person and explains what he has, if the person insists he explains, he calls me. So I feel more at ease."

"Everything on the table. We don't stop eating anything. And if someone hides it, it's worse, because it seems to pique their curiosity. I say: 'Look, don't hide it.

"Look, we always talk to him. We don't know the right way to talk, but we say: 'You've got a tummy ache. Your classmate doesn't have it, but you do. If you eat it, it'll hurt you'. And we talk and talk.

The Special Recipe Book for Phenylketonuria (Kanufre *et al.* 2001b) was published, containing recipes that the mothers themselves exchanged with each other in the SR, and is given to each new patient who arrives at the programme. All the recipes were tested and quantified in terms of yield and phe content per portion. One of the mothers revealed her opinion of the book.

> *"The book is very important, the recipes are very important. For me, when I left here with the recipe book, it was like a child getting a lollipop. Then I said: Here, people, there's food, look!*

This initiative has greatly encouraged the diversification of the diet at home, at school and at other special events. It has thus become an instrument for selecting and preparing food, often with four hands, when the child is old enough to take part in making the recipes.

Families also often try to identify foods with a lower concentration of phe to offer their children during outings away from home.

> *"We (the parents) do a little shopping for ourselves and leave one at Grandad's house."*

> *"APAE São Paulo has an experimental kitchen, and they make the food themselves and industrialise it. So you can order anything [...] via the website. They send it bySedex. There are skewers, frozen foods, savoury snacks, cakes, bread, you name it. Everything comes with the right amount of phenyl in each item. But what I can order is everything that isn't frozen, because otherwise it spoils."*

Some companies or institutions also make the products they sell to phenylketonurics available on their websites. However, because they are located outside the state, families are limited to buying only non-perishable products, but not all of them can afford them.

Considering that the SR for treatment is located in Belo Horizonte, and the city has better access to other places, one of the mothers interviewed suggested the commercialisation of special food for PKU, similar to what happens at APAE São Paulo.

> "The *staff here are very good, but I think they can still help more, in terms of providing food for the children. We can't find food in the supermarket. So it would be very nice if there was a support centre here to offer food to the children. I miss that. Even for marketing, it would be great if there was one here like there is in São Paulo, you know? It would be excellent, because access here is much easier.*

It is therefore hoped that the team will discover alternatives that will expand the range of speciality foods on offer and also make it easier to take the special formula for PKU.

Two of the mothers interviewed said they hoped that, as their children grew up, they would become more committed to the diet.

> *"When you're around seven years old, it's easier. They'll understand how to talk, how to have a dialogue, right? So, I see it like this, when they reach a certain age they won't have any difficulties, right?" ?*

> *"Because they surprise us, you know? Just as sometimes I think he's going to get dented, he's going to get upset, and he pulls it off so well that it scares me."*

In short, the progress of CD treatment is influenced by many factors. The parents' hope is that as the child matures over time, the level of awareness and autonomy for monitoring the diet will increase.

In some of the testimonies, other expectations for improving adherence to treatment were also reported. The development of a protein substitute with a better flavour, the discovery of a drug that meets the need for treatment and, who knows, the long-awaited cure?

> *"My biggest concern is that the treatment evolves quickly so that we have more options for something that tastes better. My biggest concern now is this: how he's going to accept PKU from now on."*

> *"Of course it's good to think about if a cure were discovered. If, for example, we discovered a medicine that the child could take and could eat anything."*

C. Implications of phenylketonuria for the family and social circle

A diagnosis of CD in the family can be a stressor that affects the child's normal development and the family's social relationships. The consequences extend to the family structure, requiring reorganisation to meet daily needs and care for dietary treatment, and can also affect interpersonal relationships. The burden on all family members is natural, and psychological unpreparedness for coping with CD in childhood is often identified, jeopardising the adaptation of the child and the family itself to the new situation (CASTRO; PICCININI, 2002; Silva; Corrêa, 2006).

Russel, Mills and Zucconi (1988) reported in their study that approximately 25 per cent of PKU patients suffer significant changes in their family structure due to the constant stress and need for help.

Castro et al. (2012) carried out a study in the state of Rio Grande do Sul and reported that carers need to understand the importance of their roles in their children's development so that they can stimulate them. Once again, the influence of socio-cultural factors can be seen here, as families often find it difficult to understand their role in stimulating their children.

However, the mothers interviewed reported that after the impact of the diagnosis and the start of treatment, the routine tends to be established with the child's normal development and good acceptance of the diet. At the same time, awareness of the need for appropriate treatment becomes the main objective, above all difficulties. The mothers interviewed identified feelings of fulfilment, relief, satisfaction and, above all, that every effort is worthwhile.

These results are also corroborated by the study by Perricone *et al.* (2012) which revealed that mothers of children with chronic illnesses, despite the critical situation, showed an optimistic view of managing problems with care and the ability to ask for help.

C.1 Economic implications for the family after diagnosis

The interruption of maternal labour activities is one of the important changes that can occur in the family. As well as jeopardising the budget, it can have consequences such as emotional and social damage. The reduction in family income can also threaten the adequate supply of food, not only for the child affected, but also for the other members of the household. According to Table 6.1, half of the mothers worked outside the home and eight of them (57.1%) reported an income of less than three minimum wages.

The mothers interviewed reported difficulties in reconciling work outside the home with the activities involved in caring for a child with PKU.

> *"It changed my whole life. I used to love working. After I had her and discovered this little problem, I couldn't work any more. I went into depression wanting to work. Right now I'm counting the days to travel every two months to see if I can work. Because I need to help my husband. We live on rent. We wanted a little place for her future. I've had several interviews and all that really stuck was the travelling thing. Not every employer is understanding.*

It is difficult for mothers to continue working, especially in the first year of the child's life, as appointments are very frequent during this period. However, the mother's reintegration into the labour market can occur after this period, and mothers try to use legal means such as leave, time off and holidays to take the child to all the SR appointments.

This could probably be a time of reorganisation for the family, in which they have already adapted to the situation generated by the illness. In addition to the expectation of increasing the family's income, work also brings a return to life, according to one of the mothers.

> *"I tried to come back because it occupies my mind a lot. And you don't become obsessed, connected, tuned into the phenyl, you know? If I stay (working) I don't freak out. So it's an escape valve [...]. I have someone I trust to look after my daughter. It helps.*

Awiszus and Unger (1990) also revealed in their study that one of the mothers interviewed reported that, after the diagnosis and during treatment, she felt destroyed for at least six months. She said that she was only able to cope with the diet and all those calculations because she wasn't working; otherwise, she doesn't think she would have been able to.

In social circles, especially with relatives, phenylketonurics are often pitied for having to live with such a restrictive diet. The reactions triggered by the diagnosis are often mixed with feelings of guilt and overprotection. Three of the mothers interviewed revealed their relatives' attitudes towards the child's diet.

"As much as he (the father) tries to hide it, deep down he feels very sorry for her, he keeps looking for something to give her. He always likes to go out with her, give her a popsicle. He always likes to please her, within the limits of what she can eat."

"My mother-in-law usually gives him the things he can't have. There's no point in us doing our bit at home and then they don't do it. Then I say: don't be sorry .... You have to feel sorry if he eats it".
"I've also heard other people say: '[...] I feel sorry for you. Your food is so bland, you don't have any meat'. Then I draw attention to it, I don't like it. You have to tell her that her food is good too, it's delicious.

Difficulties in imposing limits on the child or withholding food were also reported.

"[...] he comes to his grandmother: 'Oh Grandma, just give me one, it won't hurt'. He cries like that in the morning and they feel sorry for him. He comes up to his grandfather and asks him to go to the pub to buy some sweets and his grandfather takes pity and goes to hide from me. He's already throwing a tantrum, saying he's going to run away from home to buy sweets. So it's complicated.

"Now he screams at anything, he keeps screaming. Then he cries another time. Now he cries screaming, throwing tantrums. Because I say no. He doesn't care about no, he doesn't care about limits. That's the difficulty".

"My mum sometimes says to me: 'She already has this problem

Because the child already has a number of limitations, parents and relatives are reluctant to set limits and criteria for behaviour; this attitude can contribute to the child using manipulation with tricks and insistent requests for something not allowed in the diet, as well as bargaining.

Some of the mothers interviewed reported that it was also a difficult task to delegate the necessary care of a child with PKU to relatives or friends.

Sharing the care of a child with PKU is a situation that can bring insecurity to both sides.

People in the family and close social circle who aren't involved in the treatment and don't attend appointments find it harder to help with the treatment and support the child's diet. Sometimes they even offer foods that are not allowed, influencing the child's habitual consumption. This fragility can encourage treatment abandonment or neglect, since the results of poor control of blood levels of phe will only become evident, especially at school age, when children will generally have difficulty with literacy and learning. However, there were reports of family members, neighbours and friends helping with the treatment.

"All my neighbours, my family, my workplace, everyone knows about her problem. What she can eat, what she can't eat. She herself knows that she has Phenylketonuria. If I need to leave it with my mum, my sister-in-law, my brother, everyone is committed to her treatment."

It should be emphasised that the role of the family is fundamental. Sooner or later, the phenylketonuric will live with other people and will have to find the conditions to maintain treatment naturally.

Some of the mothers interviewed also reported difficulties in maintaining routines, such as supermarket shopping, travelling, going to restaurants and visiting other people.

"A woman said: 'You don't want to buy the train for the boy because you don't have any money'? I said: No. If he could eat, I would have bought it. I didn't buy it because he can't. So I'd rather stay at home and have fun with my son.

"When travelling, you have to do a lot of research about the place you're going to in order to know if you're going to be able to take part in things. So it does restrict socialising. It's difficult, because sometimes you go out and you have to leave with a huge packet. If you go to a restaurant, they won't accept you putting anything on the table that doesn't belong to the restaurant".

It's common to observe that people who don't yet know or understand the disease can cause embarrassment and conflict and influence families to isolate themselves in order to preserve the affected child.

In the study carried out by Frank, Fitzgerald and Legge (2007), the authors also reported difficulty maintaining the diet in environments surrounded by industrialised foods and in travel situations. The patients interviewed said that the hardest consequence of PKU is having to constantly think about what you can and cannot eat.

On the other hand, there were reports of mothers who managed to get round these situations, always keeping their focus on the treatment in any environment.

> *"XI visits other people's houses, goes to pizzerias, barbecues, we never stop doing anything because of this. We go out every weekend and always take what she can eat and she's always interacting with us. Everyone at the same table. She eats what she can.*

In some of the testimonies, we observed families who turn PKU into a cause for isolation; others try to overcome the disease, providing a better quality of life for the child.

Many mothers reported that they choose not to attend parties and other social events to avoid conflicts and problems in monitoring their child's diet.

> *"Within the family, I'll tell you the truth, if he went to two parties it was a lot. When I go, I take his little things. I make the special food, but he questions it too much. He eats, but I prefer to avoid it. We hardly ever go".*

> *"The different things they offer at parties, she stares and I'm afraid of watering, because they used to say that it would water, right? Then I leave."*

> *"It's difficult. Because especially at a birthday party, he already looks and really draws attention, because you see a table decorated with cake. I shouldn't, but I've already stopped going to several birthday parties because of this."*

Thus, the difficulty imposed by a diet that is so different from the one normally consumed by the population often means that phenylketonurics are isolated in an attempt not to break it. It's likely that mothers find it very uncomfortable to spend all their time watching out for dietary transgressions, as well as having to justify this control in front of other guests.

Removing the child from social activities can cause permanent exclusion, an isolation that can lead to a feeling of loneliness, which is detrimental to all aspects of the child's development. Some authors have also reported that the difference in diet creates a distinction between the individual with restrictions and others, which can lead to a lack of social acceptance, exclusion and the stigma of the disease, especially in childhood (FRANK; FITZGERALD; LEGGE, 2007; MOREIRA; DUPAS, 2006).

Other mums, however, reported going about their lives as normal, taking part in all the events, with the support of relatives and friends.

"We always take part in parties. I take her pie, her savoury snack, that little biscuit I buy in the supermarket that has zero protein. Sometimes, at the sweets table, I show her one or two sweets that she can have, fruit, jujube. What she can't have, I tell her she can't have. What am I going to do? If you can't have it, you won't eat it.

"[...] we've been with him to parties. He can see the cake, the sweets, the snacks on the table. Even if you take the snack and put it in his hand, he won't eat it.

He says it's not his. But we think he'll end up wanting it.

Families that are generally well-structured are more accepting of diagnosis and treatment and, consequently, their children are more likely to react in the same way.

C.3 Children at school

School-age phenylketonurics bring new concerns for parents and educators. The mothers revealed a lot of insecurity and anxiety about their child starting school. On the other hand, they don't want their children to be treated differently from other children.

The mothers fear that the school environment will be favourable to dietary transgressions, especially during snack time. According to the mothers' testimonies, among the doubts, the most worrying is who will control their child's diet.

It's common for children to share the food they bring for snack. In the case of school meals, most preparations are not allowed for phenylketonurics. Some examples are rice with meat, sausage with sauce, beans, popcorn, chocolate, biscuits, rice pudding and puddings.

Educators also feel under pressure and sometimes even responsible for ensuring that nothing gets out of hand while the child is in their care. The rare, little-known disease further accentuates the feeling of insecurity and fragility. Therefore, ensuring that the child is not affected by the sequelae that poor diet control can cause seems to be everyone's goal. Castro et al. (2012) found that a phenylketonuric child with regular control over the course of treatment was 3.86 times more likely to have an upper and middle QI when compared to children who were classified as having inadequate control.

In addition to the fear of transgression, the mothers reported concerns about the variety of snacks the child would be able to take to school and their efforts to come up with special recipes.

> *"My son is going to school next year. My expectation is that we don't keep putting everything the same. He might not even like having the same snack every day. I'm a bit anxious, but I'm going to have to be very calm and brave in order to make a lot of different snacks for him."*

> *"I make coxinha, pastel, cake, bread, ice cream, banana brigadeiro. He takes it well, but he gets sick very easily. He eats it a few times and doesn't want it any more. Then you have to switch to something else."*

> *"I wake up early in the morning, make snacks, bake a cake. I haven't managed to make it that marvellous, but I try and at least he can eat it. I do it, but he questions too much. We explain, explain, but he questions a lot!"*

In this study, one of the mothers reported her indignation at how her child was treated during school meals.

> "She wanted to keep him away at snack time, you know? Put him in a separate room, and I didn't think that was right. Because if he has to live with it, it has to start now."

Sometimes, the school and the teacher themselves prefer to segregate phenylketonurics in different spaces from the rest of their classmates during school.

snack. This attitude of isolation is probably more of an attempt to protect the child, to avoid food offences, rather than to discriminate against them. Unfortunately, this practice is still common and reinforces the stigma of the disease and the social exclusion of phenylketonurics.

Other situations that cause anxiety and insecurity for families and teachers are festive events at school. In order to make it possible for children to take part in these occasions, mothers have to make an extra effort to prepare alternative recipes.

"I find out what's on at school, at the party. If there's a sandwich, I make it for him. If there's snacks, we always have frozen snacks. If there's popcorn, we buy the popcorn. Cake, we take his cake.

"He eats in front of everyone, he's with everyone. I want him to take part in everything, I don't want him to be left out of anything. I get involved. On ice-cream day, I made his ice-cream. He joined the queue just like everyone else, only when it was his turn, he put his in. And off he goes, happy as a clam.

It is necessary, and certainly everyone's wish, for children to be able to take part in festive activities and accept eating what is theirs. So many mothers organise themselves to prepare special recipes for the festivities. The expectation is that phenylketonurics will be better prepared for life, as they won't be able to live in isolation. However, it is undeniable that they are attracted to the snacks and treats that other children of the same age consume, especially those publicised by the media.

Whilst on the one hand the school can be a source of concern for some families, on the other it can be a great ally in the child's treatment. Two mothers revealed a positive relationship with the school.

"There's no problem at school. She takes her snack. She snacks with everyone. These days there was a party for the teachers, so I took the (brand of product) cupcake. When the snack, the soft drink and the cake were going to be served, she only ate her snack. She couldn't eat the snacks".

"Today I have the school to help me. Both in terms of food and setting limits. I had a chat at school with the teacher and the headmistress and asked them: Please don't treat him differently, because this will reflect at home. I'll lose everything I've done. I share my burden with the school. Not the bad load, the good load, you know?

The school's integration with the family is fundamental and can become a safe haven for parents, sharing information, dividing responsibilities and including the child in all school and festive activities. Currently, at CEAPS, the pedagogue and nutritionist contact the school when the need for any intervention is identified. This communication channel has also been very useful for discussing, clarifying and seeking information about the child's behaviour and school performance.

Conclusions

The study made it possible to broaden our understanding of the psychosocial and behavioural aspects of phenylketonuric children in their environment. By expressing their anxieties and difficulties in dealing with PKU in the family dynamic, the mothers interviewed were able to reflect on the issues involved in treatment and the importance of adherence.

The transmission of the screening test result is a crucial moment that triggers the shock of having a different child, and the lack of preparation on the part of professionals to notify this change accentuates this impact.

The absence of signs of the disease in affected children undergoing regular treatment can lead to doubts about its existence, making it difficult to believe in the diagnosis and commit to treatment.

During their child's treatment, the mothers experienced feelings that are common in the process of adapting to a serious illness, such as denial, anger, depression, acceptance and hope.

The feelings experienced, especially by the parents of the affected child, are similar to those triggered by CD. The disease has no cure and will accompany the individual for their entire life, bringing up the presence of treatment and potential risks on a daily basis.

As the mother most often accompanies the child to the Referral Service and almost exclusively takes charge of the treatment, the family finds it harder to understand the disease and, in this way, can make it difficult to adhere to the diet and contribute to dietary transgressions. Considering that maternal overload is unquestionable, mothers carry the burden of greater responsibility for dietary control, favouring strain on family relationships, as well as stress, anguish and feelings of loneliness. Starting school is a second moment of tension for them. However, it has not represented a significant obstacle to maintaining the diet.

On the other hand, the mothers revealed that it was comforting to know that there is treatment for PKU and that it is available to everyone through the SUS. It is an effective treatment that allows affected children to live a normal life.

The fear of social exclusion is yet another consequence of chronic illness. Parents fear that their children won't be able to socialise, especially as they consider that food permeates a large part of social relationships. However, they hope that with the passage of time and the maturing of their children, there will be greater awareness and autonomy in monitoring their diet.

The mothers also showed interest and satisfaction when they were included in the study to talk about their feelings, emphasising the importance of sensitive listening. Establishing links and forming partnerships is one of the ways to rebuild health practices in a humanised way.

The evolution of treatment for CD is influenced by various factors and requires significant changes in the family structure. There are still many questions to be addressed regarding the repercussions of Phenylketonuria on family dynamics.

There is a fertile field of research to elucidate other issues that are essential to treatment, such as: identifying factors that can contribute to improving adherence to the diet; developing a more palatable protein substitute that is easy to handle and fractionate throughout the day; producing and identifying new industrialised quality products for PKU; widely publicising the disease to all institutional sectors and to the general population.

The results of this study provided a better understanding of the daily difficulties and challenges of living with and caring for a child with phenylketonuria. It is hoped that the information generated can contribute to a more humanised and integrated approach to Phenylketonuria, in a scenario that encourages the construction of strategies that facilitate the control of the disease, improving the quality of life of this population.

The perception of the multi-professional team on the care and treatment of Phenylketonuria

Introduction

Phenylketonuria (PKU) is an autosomal recessive genetic disease caused by the deficiency or absence of the liver enzyme phenylalanine hydroxylase (PHA), which is responsible for hydroxylating phenylalanine (phe) into tyrosine (tyr). Deficiency of this enzyme leads to an increase in blood concentrations of phe, reaching the central nervous system and causing irreversible mental retardation of varying intensity (SCRIVER; KAUFMAN, 2001).

Diagnosis should preferably be carried out in the neonatal period, before symptoms appear, since neurological damage is irreversible. Blood samples for neonatal screening should be taken between the third and fifth day of life to ensure sufficient protein intake and reduce the incidence of false-negative cases of PKU, while also allowing for early treatment (STARLING et al, 1999).

The Minas Gerais State Neonatal Screening Programme (PETN-MG) screens approximately 94% of newborns in the state and is coordinated by the Centre for Action and Research in Diagnostic Support at the Faculty of Medicine of the Federal University of Minas Gerais (NUPAD-FM-UFMG). As well as being responsible for diagnosis, it provides treatment and follow-up for patients affected by the diseases screened, through partnerships with the Hospital das Clínicas and the Municipal and State Health Departments (AGUIAR, 2004).

In Minas Gerais, PKU treatment is centralised in Belo Horizonte, at the Phenylketonuria Outpatient Clinic of the Special Genetics Service of the

UFMG Hospital das Clínicas (SEG-HC-UFMG) by a multi-professional team made up of doctors, nutritionists, nurses, psychologists, educators and social workers. Currently, 295 patients are being cared for by the Reference Service. Of these, 237 (80.3%) were diagnosed early by neonatal screening, while the other 58 (19.7%) were diagnosed late and identified for a variety of reasons, including being relatives of others screened positive for the disease or patients transferred from other neonatal screening programmes in the country.

Of all the patients seen, eight (2.7 per cent) had a Tetrahydrobiopterin (BH4) deficiency, which is responsible for more serious clinical conditions, as it alters the formation of neurotransmitters (STARLING, 2005).

The treatment of PKU is dietary and consists of a diet restricted in phe and the use of a protein substitute, free of or with a low concentration of phe, plus tyr, vitamins and mineral salts (ACOSTA; YANNICELLI, 2001; CORNEJO; RAIMAN, 2010; SHAW; LAWSON, 1994).

In most countries, including Brazil, maintaining treatment is recommended for the patient's entire life. Thus, individuals with PKU should maintain a diet restricted in phe for the rest of their lives, as its interruption is associated with a worsening of the Intellectual Quotient (QI), decreased attention and speed of information processing in adults. Furthermore, according to some studies, interrupting the diet is also related to loss of concentration, hyperactivity and irritability (FRANK; FITZGERALD; LEGGE, 2007; MACDONALD, 2010; NATIONAL INSTITUTES OF HEALTH CONSENSUS, 2001).

Despite the risks, MacDonald *et al.* (2010) reported in their study that non-compliance with treatment is universal, emphasising that any approach to improving adherence to treatment must be based on careful diagnosis of possible associated factors. The quality of the diet imposed, psychosocial factors, acceptance of the diagnosis by the family and the patient themselves, difficulties inherent to age, eating habits and lifestyle can all make it difficult to properly engage in treatment.

The dietary management of PKU is considered a successful and effective model for the treatment of an inherited metabolic disease that allows patients to develop neuropsychomotor function properly. However, it is necessary to maintain the perspective that treatments should not be based solely on long-term clinical results, but also on the life experience of people living with the disease. Research into treatment adherence, exploring this experience, has shown that professional support can be improved to better meet the needs of phenylketonurics and their families in both medical and emotional aspects (FRANK; FITZGERALD; LEGGE, 2007).

Finally, it cannot be denied that the management of chronic disease (CD) is still a challenge for professionals, often bringing up feelings of impotence and frustration, since theoretical training and the biological approach are not enough to encompass the complexity of care and treatment that requires a more accurate perception of living with the disease.

Clavreul (1983) reveals that the medical discourse dismisses elements that are of interest to the treatment; elements that are considered foreign to this discourse and at the same time singularly present. These include the various sufferings that cannot be medically justified, functional disorders, mood swings and anxieties that can be continually presented to doctors by patients, leaving them entirely disarmed by the absence of an acceptable scientific interpretation for treating them. For the author:

> *"The object of medicine is disease. An ontology that insists. The illness is a Being foreign to the patient. Its identity must be assured" (p.121).*

> *"Medical discourse essentially aims to dispossess the patient of his illness and, if possible, to rid him of it. By constituting the illness as an Entity, the doctor dispossesses the patient of it in*

An opposite movement points to the *Shared Extended Clinic,* one of the guidelines of the Humanisation Policy of the SUS, which seeks to constitute a tool for the articulation and inclusion of different approaches and disciplines, since health work distinguishes between three major areas of activity: biomedical, social and psychological (BRASIL, 2009).

The *Extended and Shared Clinic* recognises that, in a given moment and unique situation, there may be a predominance, a choice, or the emergence of one approach or theme, without this meaning the negation of others and possibilities for action. Another aspect concerns the urgent need to share health diagnoses and behaviour with users, both individually and collectively. The longer the course of treatment and the greater the need for the subject to participate and adhere to their therapeutic project, the greater the challenge of dealing with the user as a subject, seeking their participation and autonomy in their treatment. The functioning of the Reference Teams makes it possible for professionals to take direct responsibility for the care and joint construction of a Singular Therapeutic Project. The *Extended Clinic* proposal *is* based on a broader understanding of the health-disease process; the shared construction of diagnoses and therapies; the expansion of the object of work; the transformation of the means or instruments of work and support for health professionals (BRASIL, 2009).

Vieira and Lima (2002) reported that scientific and technological development has made it possible to diagnose diseases at an early stage and apply appropriate therapies. However, according to the authors, even with these advances, chronic illnesses are subject to organic, emotional and social changes that require constant care and adaptation.

Thus, considering the complexity of the subject and the need to better understand the implications of PKU, this study was proposed in order to understand the perception of the multi-professional team on the care and treatment of the affected child, as well as to identify strategies for overcoming the difficulties experienced by the team.

Method

A qualitative study was carried out, based on the testimonies of professionals working in the SR of the state of Minas Gerais on the care and treatment of children with Phenylketonuria. Considering the objectives of the study, a focus group (FG) was chosen for data collection.

The FG is a type of group interview that emphasises communication between research participants, based on topics that are provided by the researcher who guides the focus, but the data is generated by the interaction of its members (KITZINGER, 2006; RIGOTTO, 1998).

Ten professionals from different areas of knowledge who work in the reception and care of phenylketonuric patients in the SR were invited to take part in this study. The inclusion criteria were: being a professional from the Phenylketonuria Outpatient Clinic at SEG-HC/NUPAD/FM/UFMG, the Treatment Control Sector (SCT-NUPAD) and the Education and Social Support Centre (CEAPS-NUPAD) involved in the treatment of phenylketonurics. Two invited professionals did not turn up for the activity, as previously arranged. Eight took part, including paediatricians and geneticists, nutritionists, nurses, social workers, administrative assistants and technicians. The supervisor and the research author who conducted the FG were excluded.

The meeting took place in February 2013. For data collection, the dynamics were based on a pre-prepared script of five questions, based on the review of related literature, the experience acquired by the researcher at the Phenylketonuria Outpatient Clinic and in accordance with the objectives of the study (Chart 7.1).

Table 7.1 **Table 7.1 Questionnaire for the focus group**

Questions
- What has it been like caring for children with Phenylketonuria and their families?
- What is your perception of approaching parents and family members at the 1ª consultation?
- How do you perceive adherence to treatment?
- From an institutional point of view, what are the biggest difficulties that the service find and the strategies to overcome them?
- What major challenges do you identify in treatment and follow-up? of children with an early diagnosis of PKU?

Before starting the FG activities, the researcher gave a brief explanation of the study and its objectives. The use of the recording tool was explained. The Free and Informed Consent Form

The Informed Consent Form (Figure 5.3) was signed and then the participants introduced themselves.

The activity time of the FG was one hour and eighteen minutes (1:18h). The entire discussion was recorded on MP3 and the material collected on audio was transcribed in its entirety by the researcher with the help of an undergraduate student in Nutrition at UFMG, thus enabling a better understanding of the recorded content. The anonymity of the group members was preserved. To guarantee the confidentiality of the information, the participants were identified by codes (P1, P2P8   ).

To analyse the material collected, the Content Analysis technique was used, with a floating reading of all the material collected, followed by an in-depth reading (BARDIN, 2011). The data was grouped by theme and, in a classification process, the main categories were identified. Subsequently, the final analysis was carried out, with treatment and interpretation of the results obtained. Throughout the analysis process, confrontation with data from the literature and the researchers was carried out as a triangulation strategy.

This study was approved by the Research Ethics Committee of the Federal University of Minas Gerais (COEP-UFMG), process CAAE 0525.0.203.000-09.

Results and discussion

The length of time the participants had been working in the state's SR ranged from one to eighteen years. Six of them are senior professionals and two are mid-level professionals.

Analysis of the focus group with the multi-professional team

Analysing the transcribed material made it possible to identify three main categories with their subdivisions, as shown in Table 7.2.

Table 7.2 Categories and subcategories identified in the focus group

Categories	Sub-categories
A. 0 start of treatment	A.1 Reception of families at the Centre for Education and Social Support (CEAPS) A.2 Impressions of the first visit to the Phenylketonuria Outpatient Clinic
B. The work of the multi-professional team	8.1 In the Phenylketonuria Outpatient Clinic 8.2 At the Centre for Education and Social Support (CEAPS)
C. Difficulties experienced	C.1 In the Reference Service C.2 In the PKU child's municipality of origin C.3 At school C.4 Adherence to treatment C.5 Strategies and challenges

A. The start of treatment

The professionals who took part in the FG reported on the importance of welcoming patients and their families and their impressions of the first day of care. At the first appointment, families arrive very anxious, both for the news and for the quick and necessary referral to the SR, whenever a suspected diagnosis of PKU arises.

Araújo *et al.* (2013) also revealed that the family's first encounter with the health service of reference is fundamental for professionals and families seeking a strong ally in coping with the disease.

A.1 Welcoming families at

Centre for Education and Social Support (CEAPS)

One of the participants in the FG tried to describe the type of approach that is taken during the first visit to the SR.

> *"This welcome is in the sense of finding out how she came, how she's feeling. It's more superficial, right? [...] And from this welcome we can see some of the issues that the family brings, even from an emotional point of view."*

The first contact takes place at CEAPS, right after the blood test, where parents and other family members have the opportunity to obtain initial information about the disease. At this point, it is already possible to see the emotional issues that afflict families.

One of the professionals recounted his feelings at the first reception.

> *"I always want to welcome them, especially because we're there at CEAPS. We realise how much these families need a different kind of listening ear, information. [...] We are their mainstay, their support. So I feel a great responsibility towards them.*

The need for differentiated listening and the support given to families throughout treatment are implicit in the team's sense of commitment and responsibility. The bond gradually established between professionals, patients and families can become a great ally in treatment.Bergman, Lewiston and West (1979) reported the importance of early assessment of chronic paediatric patients and their families, with a view to selecting appropriate interventions for these families. They consider it of paramount importance to minimise feelings of helplessness, dependence and isolation during treatment. They also emphasise the need to mobilise resources, encourage families to bring up their problems and share their experiences with other families.

The professionals reported their impressions of the first contact with the families and their reactions to the SR.

> *"I've always noticed that there's a lot of shock on the part of the family. We avoid giving them all the information when they first contact us."*
> *"The family doesn't know what it is, they don't know what Phenylketonuria is."*

Parents are notified of the change in the screening test in their municipality of origin. The type of approach that is taken and the first information about the disease can interfere with how the family will deal with the diagnosis and treatment, especially in the first few months of the child's life. There are always reactions of shock, fright, denial and even resistance to the diagnosis, which can extend throughout treatment.

One of the professionals taking part in the FG recounted his experience during his first consultation with the family at the Phenylketonuria Outpatient Clinic.

> *"We explain that it's a genetic disease, [...] that the parents are carriers of a mutation, but that they're not sick and that it's an evolutionary thing, a natural thing. And then the parents ask: 'Is there a cure'? And we say: There is no cure, just as no genetic disease has a cure, but there is a way to treat it [...] to prevent mental retardation from developing".*

At the outpatient clinic, the first medical consultation is made by the geneticist with the aim of clarifying the disease and treatment, as well as carrying out genetic counselling. Although the first reception takes place at CEAPS, it is at the consultation with the geneticist that the diagnosis is finalised. Despite the impact of the diagnosis, with each appointment parents feel more confident about the treatment and the team. However, the unexpected diagnosis brings up several common feelings experienced by the families, as some of the professionals told us.

"They can often be really angry. Anger at us, even at the boy. Guilt. What I did, what I didn't do. We explain to them that this is normal and that it can happen."

"[...] many mums blame themselves for having the child. Sometimes they even think it's something they ate that's affected the child."

"I see that when the family's reaction is delayed, it will have repercussions on the adolescent's behaviour. So we see how the family understands the illness will have repercussions in adolescence and perhaps throughout their lives."

As well as the ever-present fright and shock, other feelings arise, such as anger and guilt. These are common and expected reactions when faced with the prospect of CD, which is likely to have lifelong repercussions.

B. Multi-professional team performance

2.1 In the Phenylketonuria Outpatient Clinic

One of the professionals reported his perception of the follow-up by the geneticist throughout the treatment, since the proposed genetic approach is carried out on the day of the first consultation.

"[...] from time to time I think it's worth revisiting this (genetic) consultation. You get it the first time and then you end up losing contact".

Reinforcement of the need for good control of blood levels of Phe throughout the life of the phenylketonuric should take place. Fiese and Everhart (2006) suggest that cohesive team management strategies with families can promote long-term adherence to treatment.

One of the participants recounts the sensitisation and feelings of solidarity and affection unleashed among professionals, patients and their families.

> *"We become very sensitised to the issue of the disease. And after all these years, we really become a family, don't we? The families come to have a great deal of trust in us and we come to have a great deal of affection for them."*

On the other hand, conflicting feelings are also expressed, according to one of the professionals.

> *"Often the family rejects the team, despite their trust. There are those who hate us. They hate us in the sense of: 'You brought me the disease. You gave me the news. You gave me the diet. You're after me'. Everything is our fault. So you have to be able to deal with that too.*

Despite the trust, there are families who maintain a resistance and even rejection and anger towards some members of the team.
Even if these attitudes can be understood, they still cause discomfort and sometimes embarrassment during the appointments. These feelings are also described by Kubler-Ross (2000) at the time of diagnosis and while living with the illness, especially chronic illness.

Some professionals reported their difficulties with certain families and that sometimes a feeling of helplessness arises.

> *"As a professional, I often try to believe all the time that the treatment is effective. But of course we often get discouraged by*

The feeling of powerlessness often frightens professionals, especially when the expected adherence to treatment does not occur. This non-adherence can be related to inadequate control of blood levels of phe, absenteeism from appointments and dietary transgressions. However, it is necessary to gather strength and a lot of courage to try to uncover, understand and seek solutions to the structural problems faced by families, beyond the diagnosis; and even to mobilise resources to reach patients and carers.

In the study carried out by Silva *et al.* (2010), the authors reported that when family dynamics were already conflictual before the onset of CD, it became an additional stress factor in the family environment, thus demanding much more of its members.

According to the guidelines of the *Extended and Shared Clinic,* the more the illness is understood and correlated with life, the less likely it is to become a problem for the health service alone. In this sense, it is important to listen to and welcome all the complaints and feelings experienced by users, and that bonds and affections can be explored. Both professionals and users, whether they realise it or not, place different affections on each other. This helps them to better understand themselves and each other, increasing the chance of helping the sick person to gain more autonomy and cope with their illness. It is important to emphasise that guilt and fear should not be used as allies. Guilt paralyses, generates resistance and can humiliate. It's more productive to try to build a therapeutic proposal that is agreed with the user and for which they take co-responsibility. Dialogue and information are good tools for presenting the possible risks, so that the user can discuss them and negotiate with the team on how to proceed. Finally, illness cannot be the only concern in life. Life is broader than the means people find to keep themselves healthy (BRASIL, 2009).

On the other hand, the integration of the team and the exchange of experiences between the professionals who work in the NUPAD sectors were also emphasised in some reports.

> *"Sometimes the team itself notices some characteristic of the child that isn't normal and goes to the doctor, makes a referral."*

> *"I think that the people who work at the outpatient clinic don't have as much contact with the municipality and [...] they expose the family's difficulties [...]. My contact isn't directly with the family. It's more with the Health Unit [...] And so, the exchange of information between us professionals, I think that's quite interesting. We can see both sides, the family's side and the municipality's side.*

> *"I'd even like to stress the importance of the team being cohesive, having a good dialogue, us always having meetings [...]. This is important, because the team gives us support [...] even from an emotional point of view, for our professional work. I think that today we're well in tune, well connected [...]. All of us in the service are winners, and certainly the families and patients."*

> *"We saw how important the multi-professional team is, that it's not just the outpatient clinic at Fenil. There's a whole network for protecting and sheltering these families that will take them through this suffering."*

The exchange of knowledge makes it possible to capture the different perspectives of each member of the team, which allows for a broader and, at the same time, unique observation of each patient and their family. The questions that come up in the weekly pre-ambulatory meetings serve as a guide to help with the care and dialogue with the patient's family.

family, solving problems and making referrals to other specialities. The team also functions as a professional support strategy in dealing with adverse situations, a kind of strengthening that, in a chain, can enliven the relationship with family members and patients.

Team meetings are considered privileged spaces for dialogue in order to articulate the various intervention resources available to the team, and there needs to be a climate in which everyone has the right to a voice and an opinion. As the team realises its limits and difficulties, it can ask for help. When there is an interest in a particular topic, the capacity for learning is greater. Therefore, this is potentially an excellent space for exchange and learning, for ongoing training (BRASIL, 2009).

Today, the multi-professional team is an undeniable and necessary reality in all areas where actions are taken to improve people's quality of health and life. The question is how to make it work in a homogeneous, democratic, aggregative and co-operative way. Teamwork can function as a device for finding creative and constructive ways of solving complex problems, as long as the specificity of each professional is respected and the common areas are supported by the practices and knowledge of all professionals.

The *Expanded Clinic* then proposes that health professionals develop the ability to help people not only to fight disease, but to transform themselves, so that the disease, even if it is a limit, does not prevent them from experiencing other things in their lives (BRASIL, 2009).

The NUPAD has several sectors working as a network, thus ensuring a well-articulated process between them and the patients' municipalities of origin. This integration optimises the active search, collection and timely processing of blood samples. The connection between CEAPS and the Phenylketonuria Outpatient Clinic also makes it possible to provide more effective care.

Another issue reported in the FG was the professional development of the team.

> *"The professionals wanted to specialise a little more in the disease, precisely to try to manage the treatment in the best possible way. We always try to study so that these families receive more qualified care from us*

The growing number of patients, the diversity of cases and the variety of problems faced by families and their children with PKU are placing new demands on the team's knowledge. For this reason, professionals have sought further training in specialisation, master's and doctoral courses, developing studies on the disease, treatment and knowledge of the factors that may interfere with adherence.

2.2 At the Centre for Education and Social Support (CEAPS)

On consultation days, some activities take place systematically at CEAPS during the morning shift, after blood collection. Some of the participating professionals reported their impressions.

> *"There are some who, when they see the toys there, go crazy. Because most of them (...) don't have what they have there at home. There's even one who says: 'Wow, I love coming to Belo Horizonte. So they spend the morning playing in the toy library. [...] because since they're staying all day, there's an activity for them to do.*

The pedagogue's work at CEAPS is recent and is a proposal to work in non-school spaces, more specifically in the area of hospital pedagogy, with the aim of sharing and dialoguing with the knowledge of other areas of activity such as medicine, nursing, nutrition, psychology and social work, mediated with the educational field. The playroom is one of the recreational activities run by the pedagogue for patients waiting to be seen in the outpatient clinic, which not only provides entertainment but also allows them to socialise. The professionals who took part in the GF recognised that the strategy is a very attractive differential for the children.

Another activity mentioned by the professionals was operative groups with families. These are held weekly with a planned frequency and cover topics that are either free or on demand.

> *"[...] we're also doing operative groups. Each week we work on a theme and there are also free themes that families bring and discuss with us."*

The organisation of groups as a form of collective care for the population has become increasingly common in health services. The theoretical framework most used in this practice is that of Pichón-Rivière, an Argentinian psychoanalyst and doctor, who defines an operative group as a collective learning process: **a group of people linked together in a potential space for individual transformation, through a group experience that encourages participants to adopt an investigative attitude, transforming this learning into change.** According to Soares and Ferraz (2007), these groups are generally organised according to the type of illness, age and other criteria. The benefits of this type of care include: greater optimisation of work with fewer individual consultations; the client's active participation in the educational process and the involvement of the team of professionals with the client. The authors also emphasise that it is essential for health professionals to discuss and learn about collective phenomena, in order to understand the theoretical foundations of group dynamics and broaden their view of the group.

In this study, one of the professionals revealed that the momentary interruption of these groups caused a pent-up demand among families.

> *"There was a transition period in which we were unable to hold these groups and now we're resuming them [...]. So I can see that there is a pent-up demand. These families are bringing a lot of interesting questions, not just about the specific treatment, but about their day-to-day life, their routine. So this dialogue is interesting because many families leave feeling relieved in some way. So these groups are being productive. This has been happening at CEAPS and I think it's a job that we can do to add to all of our services.*

The resumption of activities, which takes place in parallel with the playroom, has enabled families to bring up many important issues. Situations that are often experienced by other people who are there, and that can alleviate the seriousness of the problem or, perhaps, find a solution through joint discussion. Despite this, there are complaints about the absence of the clinical team in these activities, as reported by one of the participants.

> *"The operative groups we've been running at CEAPS, I think we even need a little more participation from the outpatient professionals. Going to the geneticist, one day going to the paediatrician, there are other issues that mothers have a lot of doubts about and everything. The very issues of nutrition, breastfeeding [...]. So I think this kind of information is really interesting.*

The presence of members of the clinical care team has been requested as demands arise in the various areas of activity that need to be addressed. It can be seen that doubts about the disease or talking about it is not limited to outpatient care. Those involved seem to have a recurring need to bring up the subject, showing that the disease goes beyond the reach of institutions, where it is socially permitted to be experienced.

The expansion of the Neonatal Screening Programme and the growth of the team also brought some difficulties, according to three professionals.

"The programme covers the whole of Minas Gerais, various cultural levels. So you get reactions from every possible family. [...] often the city of origin is very precarious and even in the most advanced cities, not even the professionals themselves are able to give initial information about what Phenylketonuria might be. So sometimes even the doctor doesn't know how to approach a child with Phenylketonuria."

"The team grew and so did the number of patients. Then the difficulties started to appear in relation to understanding Phenylketonuria itself. [...] Sometimes, in this paternalistic position, we end up taking autonomy away from the child themselves. The professional ends up taking away a bit of autonomy and reinforcing the role of mother, right? So the professional often ends up slipping into this as well".

"Some time ago, contact was made directly with families to talk about appointments, to ask for tests. So I think this has also made the family feel more comfortable.
settled down a bit. It's what he said: 'In the beginning, the programme was very paternalistic'

Neonatal Screening in the state has grown in complexity over the twenty years of its existence. The initial paternalistic approach to providing care made patients and their families dependent and passive. As the SR has restructured itself to meet new demands and improved work processes, this practice has been avoided. It is expected that the individual involved in the treatment should take ownership of it and achieve their independence on their own and, with autonomy, exercise their rights and responsibilities.

If, on the one hand, the service grew in scope over the years of treatment, families became accustomed to the comforts it offered. There was a certain informality which, on the one hand, brought families closer together, but on the other, made them dependent, sharing the responsibility for adherence to phenylketonuric treatment with third parties or attributing it to them.

The prospect of organising the flow was also commented on by the professionals.

> *"The issue of decentralisation that we talk about so much, when are we going to do that?"*

> *"I also think, on the other hand, that the team perhaps doesn't have the legs and the structure for so much."*

The centralisation of SR treatment in Belo Horizonte is a further aggravating factor when it comes to the municipalities paying for the transport costs of patients and companions. Partial decentralisation of PKU treatment is a proposal in the making. Initially, this process will require additional professional efforts, which would imply greater involvement on the part of municipalities, patients and their families. At the end of its implementation, it is hoped that the quality of treatment will be maintained, with more adequate monitoring of patients, enabling, in addition to rationalising resources for the municipalities involved, a better quality of life for phenylketonurics and their families.

The SCT is responsible for contacting the municipalities to schedule appointments and identify the reasons for absences. It also requests that families be accompanied at home whenever necessary and reinforces the importance of making referrals to specialities possible. This form of communication has progressively consolidated the link between health centres and families. The TCS professionals who work directly with the health services in the municipalities reported their perceptions of the measures taken to improve communication between them.

> *"In the past, the units didn't even know the patient existed. Now, when we call to discuss an appointment, they even know who the patient is."*

> *"When the last three consecutive tests are altered, we contact them and ask them to do an active search. We ask them to look at everything. Ask the school how it is*
> *what the follow-up is. If there are any delays, if there aren't. [...]Then the unit gets back to us and says: 'Wow, but this family is so complicated, it's so difficult'. Then we go and say: Here, you can't refer them to psychology, can you? To see a psychologist, a neurologist, a cardiologist too, in the case of children who are obese. So we already ask the unit to monitor the patient as a whole, not just one disease, but to look at their whole situation. The patient and the family.*

In his testimony, one of the professionals recounted his experience of the need for the psychologist to always be present and available for appointments.

> *"When there was a psychologist who went to the outpatient clinic, who worked with these families, or even in the overload test, there was a greater demand from the families. At least they would come in and say: 'I need to speak to the psychologist'. Then there was the professional and they came. Now they know there isn't one. But there is demand [...]. We can already see that that person has a demand for psychology. There's a huge demand.*

For a long time, there was an interruption in psychology counselling and, as a result, a loss of reference for families and patients who were looking for a different kind of listening. As a result, many demands came to other professionals who, most of the time, despite listening and welcoming, were unable to provide proper care.

WEGLAGE *et al.* (2000) reported that there may be an increase in the frequency of psychosocial maladjustments in paediatric patients with chronic illness. For this reason, the authors suggest that PKU treatment should include psychosocial support not only for patients, but also for their families.

The centralised care model in Belo Horizonte has made it difficult for the municipality to connect with the patients who live there, and for them to learn about PKU. The professionals who took part in the FG revealed the consequences of the poor relationship with the Health Unit (UBS).

> *"There is still resistance from some families to creating a bond with the health unit. Most of them have a better financial situation".*

> *"We're seeing that municipalities are calling us more now to ask about collection guidelines, how it's done, how it works. At least I've noticed that there's more demand from the municipalities for treatment and follow-up."*

> *"There are a lot of issues that really come down to primary care. But there are some who want to talk to us, I think more to validate something."*

In general, when families are resistant to using the UBS, there are difficulties in monitoring treatment, overloading the SR, especially the Phenylketonuria Outpatient Centre.

On the other hand, although it's a minority, there are some families who don't need medical care at the SR because they already have a private paediatrician.

> *"[...] There are some who refuse to be seen by us because they already have a private paediatrician, but there are very few of them."*

Another difficulty in the municipality of origin of the child with PKU was pointed out by the professionals.

"I think one of the problems that interferes with adherence to treatment is the issue of TFD (treatment away from home). Patients don't come to their appointments because they can't get proper transport, because the journey is long, uncomfortable and the cars aren't equipped to travel with these patients. Municipalities that have difficulty getting the patient to travel make them miss appointments several times, interfering with the control of Phenylketonuria."

One of the most frequent reasons for absenteeism is the release of Out-of-Home Treatment (OHT), a benefit granted to patients who need treatment outside the municipality where they live. This problem is being minimised by a measure that has been adopted, as reported by two participants.

"0 absenteeism has decreased a lot, because we call [...] to let them know and they usually ask the municipality to give us feedback that they've notified the family. Then they confirm that the family will be coming to the appointment."

"There are families who come, who get the TFD. But we see reports of problems with the ambulance, the ambulance is not in an adequate state of repair, the driver sometimes makes many journeys and is tired to come, and we know that Minas Gerais is very big. There are families who travel eight, nine, ten kilometres. hours. Families are missing out because this service is not being provided properly."

The routine established by the SCT to confirm the scheduling of appointments and to promptly seek out the reasons for missed appointments with the municipalities has contributed to a reduction in absenteeism.

According to one of the participating professionals, when the municipality has difficulties transporting all the patients, sometimes phenylketonurics end up being passed over for others, since those with an early diagnosis and regular treatment don't show signs of the disease.

C.3 Difficulties at school

School performance is always a concern for parents and care staff.

One of the professionals reported his feeling of powerlessness in the face of the families, since the medical discourse about the possibility of neurological damage is far removed from their reality because they can't find any objective signs of illness in their child.

Since there is nothing concrete that could serve as a warning of the child's possible cognitive losses, systematic monitoring of neuropsychomotor development could shed more light on the child's development before he reaches school age. The prospect of a referral to APAE makes the situation more desperate, perhaps because the possibility of mental retardation is realised.

Many parents also didn't have the opportunity to study and, in principle, don't recognise the importance of education for their children's future. In this sense, the professionals reported that there may be a lack of encouragement to study in the family. However, a lack of study in school does not mean a lack of education and continued learning. Phenylketonurics may have more modest aspirations for their future, different from what the team imagines is best for them.

> *"The parents are sometimes illiterate. So we don't have the encouragement. There are boys who have normal exams and so on, the other day one turned to me and I said: 'Do you want to carry on studying'? He's graduating from the eighth grade. He's he said: 'No. I want to stay in the fields, to do the work with my father'."*

> *"We have a case of a child who is now a teenager, almost a woman, who could write her name when she was six. A very humble father and mother, alcoholic parents, a very serious social situation. Her exams were terrible. Then I came in and said to her mum: 'If she carries on with this bad test, she won't be able to do well at school'. Then her mother turned to me and said: 'Her father and I are illiterate, she can write her name. That's too good' [...]".*

The school doesn't seem to be prepared to accept individuals who are different from the rest. Even if it understands this need, it is often unable to provide differentiated care. Some of the FG participants questioned the reception of phenylketonurics at school and their social inclusion.

> *"Talking to the canteen worker, talking to the teacher herself and the question of the social insertion of the child at lunchtime: 'It's not to be separated'. That's the guidance we give.*

> *"If the general population can be accepted at school, including other chronic illnesses, Down's Syndrome, why can't phenylketonurics who have a problem be accepted? For example, that boy with a late diagnosis said he didn't like going to APAE anymore, he wants to go to school because he wants to learn to read and write. And he has the right. He has this goal and APAE says he can't do it. He can write his name, he can see syllables. So he needs to be included in school."*
> *"We're even looking at inclusion in the labour market."*

It is often observed that phenylketonurics are isolated in order to preserve them, especially in terms of diet. Considering that school has a marked influence on people's lives, adverse events can result in significant intellectual, emotional and social damage.

One of the FG participants reported his optimism at the possibility of developing psycho-pedagogical work with these children.

> *"I had a nice surprise the other day with two new professionals who were very welcoming to the question of psychology and pedagogy. It was something I was very concerned about, something we had always talked about. The inclusion of these children in society. Because some of them have limitations that sometimes their families don't understand and say: 'Oh, he's ill, so he can't do this, he can't do that'."*

C.4 Difficulties in adhering to treatment

Ongoing treatment requires a strict routine, not only in terms of diet, but also frequent visits to the SR and monthly blood tests in the municipality of origin, from the second year of life onwards.

Initially, despite the impact of the PKU diagnosis, treatment is simpler, especially in the first year of life. Because at this stage the child is totally dependent and the diet is

relatively simple. As the child gradually acquires autonomy, they are encouraged to eat other foods that are common to the population but forbidden to phenylketonurics. One of the participants revealed his perception of the difficulty of adhering to PKU treatment.

> *"There's great difficulty in adhering to treatment. [...] we see from the stages of life, from clinical observation that up to the age of one or two, they have very good adherence. In the first year, there's a very recent diagnosis in the minds of families, irreversible mental retardation. The diet is much more relaxed,*

According to official statistics, only around 50 per cent of patients with chronic diseases in developed countries adhere to appropriate therapy in the long term. It is therefore necessary to carry out an accurate assessment of adherence behaviour in order to plan effective and efficient treatment (WHO, 2003).

One of the phenylketonurics interviewed in Frank's study; Fitzgerald; Legge (2007) claimed to always explain her situation when in social circumstances as a way of not appearing rude due to the lack of food options during events. However, other interviewees reported eventually transgressing the diet when people's comfort and feelings are at stake. Burgard (2007) reports that care must be taken not to underestimate the difficulties of adherence. The author also emphasises in his study that patients need to be supported and not punished, and professionals need to be trained in adherence.

Some professionals highlighted difficulties with family members in accepting the diagnosis.

The family's resistance to accepting the diagnosis of PKU contributes to poor adherence to treatment. Furthermore, it seems that the longer this denial lasts, the negative repercussions for the affected individual are magnified.

Smith; Breasley; Aeds (1990) in their study on intelligence and dietary treatment in PKU reported that the data suggests that many children treated early continue to suffer a mild degree of neurological damage, due to the difficulties in fully controlling the metabolic abnormality. This further emphasises the need for ongoing treatment with good adherence to diet and good control of blood levels of phe.

From some of the reports, a positive aspect emerged in the FG. The professionals realised that when families have the opportunity to see the effectiveness of treatment in older phenylketonurics, they are more encouraged to follow the treatment.

> *"In the outpatient clinic, both the negative and positive aspects of the disease will be addressed. We think it's more positive when they see an older phenylketonuric. When they see that the treatment really works. This is very consoling for them".*

Another challenge reported by the professionals was the teenager with Phenylketonuria.

> *"This adolescent with Phenylketonuria, I think we had to take a different look at it, because it's going to be new for everyone, right? When they become teenagers, they have their own knowledge, they can choose things. How are we going to deal with the issue of pregnancy, when these children are now grown up and have free will?*

> *"We grew up with these kids. [...] Do we nutritionists address the issue of sexuality? Does it fall within our remit? Regardless of who the most appropriate professional is, we have to talk about it, because we feel insecure, we want these kids to take care of themselves. Parents are also very insecure about adolescence. I think that now we have to come up with more direct, objective and rapid strategies for this".*

Adolescence is marked by a tumultuous phase of rapid and intense transformations. This passage does not take place in a constant and progressive manner, but rather with advances and regressions, and its duration is determined by the passage of time or age (CARVAJAL, 2001). The emotional characteristics, behavioural manifestations and social adaptation of adolescents depend on social and cultural relationships, which require care in any situation. The process of adolescence experienced by individuals who already live with CD can become significantly more difficult and complex, especially when it involves severe dietary restrictions. Frank, Fitzgerald and Legge (2007) reported in their study that sharing food can be a great symbol of relationships, friendship, trust and even intimacy. Because of this, in some situations the act of refusing some food can mean denying intimacy or creating a feeling of hostility.

Expanding the clinic means increasing the autonomy of the user of the health service, the family and the community. The *Extended and Shared Clinic* favours the integration of a team of health workers from different areas, in search of care and treatment according to each case, with the creation of a bond with the user. The individual's vulnerability and risk are taken into account and treatment is carried out not only based on the knowledge of clinical specialists, but also takes into account the history of the person being cared for (BRASIL, 2009).

The SR team recognises that they had to learn to deal with the new demands of adolescence and, at various times, felt insecure about their approach. Adolescence with PKU brings new perspectives, demanding alternatives for living with permanent treatment and, at this stage of life, adolescents may feel even more different from the group to which they belong. This reality leads parents and professionals to look for a way to get closer, to listen and be listened to by phenylketonurics, in other words, it's important to create favourable conditions to deal with this period.

Ferreira *et aL,* (2013) reported that professionals who work with adolescents must be prepared to address emotional issues for preventive, diagnostic or therapeutic purposes. Risk-taking behaviour in adolescence is common and has social, organic and emotional consequences, which are aggravated in countries like Brazil by the high level of social exclusion. The authors also recommend some points to facilitate the relationship with the adolescent, such as confidentiality, knowing how to listen and spending more time with the adolescent.

Moreira and Dupas, 2006, carried out a study on the coexistence of children and adolescents with type 1 diabetes and reported that these individuals, when compared to a control group, showed low self-esteem. The authors suggest that it is necessary to understand their behaviours, fears and desires in order to support them in the various areas of this experience, which mainly encompasses the physical, emotional and social. The study also revealed that the difficulties and conflicts between parents and teenagers are related to the former's focus on the future, while teenagers are fixated on the present.

According to international literature (ACOSTA *et aL,* 2003; CRONE *et aL,* 2005), adherence to treatment seems to decline with age. However, in the study by Nalin (2010), older patients were classified as adherent to treatment, in relation to plasma phe in the last year. The same was true of patients with a late diagnosis of PKU. Recent data from European treatment centres also suggest that adherence is improving among adolescents (MACDONALD, 2010). One of the participants in this study also reported his perception of this issue.

> *"In adolescence, the impression I get is that there's an improvement. I think it's the teenager's own responsibility. Not all of them, either, but it's because of life goals. I see that in adolescence they seem to take up treatment again after a period when everyone has a say in their diet. So one of the things we've*

been thinking about working on is precisely that, the adolescent's autonomy, so that he can go on a diet and take responsibility for himself. Because until then, everyone has owned them, right? It's the health professional, it's the parents, it's the family [...]".

If, on the one hand, adolescence brings a series of expectations, doubts and difficulties in living and coping with this phase, on the other hand, we realise that this period can be an opportunity to take charge of one's own life, improving adherence to treatment with a view to a more promising future.

It is common to observe that people generally think of a promising future for young people when they graduate from university. Care should be taken to ensure that this life expectancy does not extend generally to phenylketonurics who adhere well to treatment with adequate control of blood levels of Phe. Personal aspirations are inherent to each individual and can be influenced by social issues, supported by the environment in which they live, family experience and structure, as well as by encouraging their children.

Two of the participants reported what they perceive as the expectations of parents, educators and professionals who accompany PKU patients.

"We have some teenagers with early diagnosis who are studying law, engineering. There's one who has already graduated in Accounting. There are even some going to university who didn't have an early diagnosis."

"But I often see a lack of motivation to go on to higher education, sometimes because of the socio-economic level itself, [...] a very modest goal for the family in relation to their lives. Now, this could come down to the social issue itself, where they live. So I don't know if this has to do specifically with Phenylketonuria, with the difficulty of understanding or with something related to that."

In the professionals' perception, the testimonies show that

phenylketonurics expect that, through treatment, they will be able to experience autonomy in life, including having the right to submit to the hardships of life. A normal life (emphasis added), not necessarily beautiful, perfect or devoid of suffering.

In the study carried out by Simon *et al.* (2008), on the assessment of quality of life and description of sociodemographic factors in adolescents and young adults with PKU, the authors concluded that PKU does not significantly deteriorate quality of life when compared to control subjects in the same age group. However, they revealed that phenylketonurics have a tendency to

develop less or delayed autonomy, with a reduced likelihood of forming a normal adult relationship.

C.5 Strategies and challenges

Phenylketonuria is still little known. It is believed that increased knowledge about the disease, its etiology, detection and treatment could demystify it. Institutions should be better adapted to fulfil their role, not only in the area of formal education, but also in the formation of the individual as a citizen, with their guaranteed rights to come and go, to choose their own path.

The team's professionals suggested some strategies to improve knowledge about the disease.

> *"I think Phenylketonuria should be publicised, both in the Basic Units and in the media, because many people have no idea what it is and how difficult the treatment is, nor do they understand it."*

> *"I think we should make more use of the media that exist, because Minas Gerais is the size of France, 853 municipalities, with all the cultural diversity we have. Many have access to the internet. Teenagers love the internet. You have the letter, the booklet, but there are those who can't read, but listen to television*

Frank; Fitzgerald; Legge (2007) also reported that healthcare professionals can reduce the anxieties and uncertainties of their patients by making it easier and easier for them to feel at ease.

disseminating information about the disease, with the internet being a good medium for this.

Several professionals emphasised that the recent decentralisation of the distribution of the special formula for PKU could strengthen the family's bond with the UBS.

"I believe that the upcoming decentralisation of PKU will increase this bond and make the municipality get to know the patient. Test results are also being sent to the health unit so that it can pass them on to the family."

"I believe that with the decentralisation of the special formula, the link has increased, because we're already getting a lot of calls from the municipalities asking: 'Look, the mother came here to see me, and I don't know what this is, I don't know how it is'. I received a call from a nutritionist asking about the diet. So she wanted to know what phenyl is like. What you have to do. If she has to prescribe a diet or not. So I think it's really bringing the family into contact with the health unit".

"The programme was very paternalistic. So today there is a deconstruction of this paternalism. I think we've reached the point of reviewing it. Trying to do what the SCT and NUPAD believe is best, which is to connect these families. According to the SUS guidelines, these patients should be linked to the Basic Health Unit. Even because we know that it is the duty of the UBS to monitor the health of these patients. You formalise a service and attest to the principles of the SUS by linking the family within the normal flow of primary care at the UBS."

The distribution of the special formula for PKU currently dispensed by the Minas Gerais State Health Department to the municipality

could improve the link between patients and their health centre, since the latter, which is also involved in the process, becomes co-responsible for releasing them to users. This distribution was carried out by the NUPAD until the beginning of 2013 and decentralisation was necessary to bring it into line with the regulations.

This initiative also helps to break down the paternalism of care.

One of the professionals recognised that the TCS's frequent contact with the BHU strengthens the bond with patients and their families.

> *"I think that contact with the unit, since the unit doesn't see the phenyl patient as a patient with a chronic illness, strengthens (the bond). Because so many times we call: 'But have you checked? Have you looked? We end up insisting so much that the individual says: 'OK, the boy who has Phenylketonuria? I know what it is'. They end up getting to know the patient and adhering to it. There are some who say: 'But again'? 'Yes, again, you're going to do an active search for me and give me feedback'. I think that's how we strengthen the bond.*

The professionals confirm that another important aspect of strengthening the bond is the referral of patients for consultations in the various specialities.

> *"I think the most important thing is that the municipality is the main executor of SUS activities. It's the municipality that's responsible for all the individual's treatment. So this link with the municipality has to be strengthened, with the health professional, with the nurse on the team. That team is linked, the one who is the carer, because it will be easier for them to receive treatment there. That's what the treatment is, it's speech therapy, sometimes physiotherapy, neuro. Here it's much more difficult. So there has to be this flow, closer to the municipality."*

The SR usually makes the requests for inter-consultations. Families also sometimes request specialised consultations, but there are difficulties with referrals and doubts about where to direct them. In Belo Horizonte, there are major bottlenecks when it comes to booking appointments. What's more, families who live outside the capital and the metropolitan region will certainly face difficulties travelling. Once again, there is a need for this link and for patients to be more closely monitored in their municipality of origin.

According to the professionals, the decentralisation of PKU treatment and follow-up is one of the service's goals, and it is likely that the state and municipalities will incur lower treatment costs; this way, it is believed that families will have more peace of mind in terms of travelling and the time spent on periodic consultations.

> *"I think decentralisation will help a lot with adherence to treatment, because you'll have a professional closer to you. Of course, there will also have to be a team close by to make all the referrals. I think these kids have serious dental problems. When the team gets involved with that child in the municipality, it's much easier to send them to a psychiatrist. There are late-onset children who need neurology, psychiatry and other professionals. I believe that with this support from the municipality we might get a better response. And we would act as a reference for the health professionals in the municipalities."*

Decentralisation will also make it possible for phenylketonurics and their families to receive clinical, nutritional, psychological and social care in their own municipality or in a hub municipality in their region. This initiative will undoubtedly further strengthen the bond between phenylketonurics in the municipality, as well as speeding up and facilitating referrals to specialities whenever necessary.

Expanded accountability for primary care has been discussed in the national debate. Its strengthening has been valued as a central strategy for building the SUS and recent guidelines highlight its role as a communication centre for thematic networks for comprehensive care (CECÍLIO *et al.*, 2012).

The active participation of the school in the child's treatment is fundamental to the child's development. One of the participants reported a recent intervention with schools.

"[...] now we have the pedagogue, who is making contact with the school, talking to the headmaster, the teacher. We're putting together a kit to send to the schools along with a letter, to talk about the team's perceptions, because of this boy's tests. So we're going to see what the school can do to help that boy.

Actions that allow the SCT to liaise, by means of reports on the progress of the child's treatment and follow-up and other clarifications, can contribute to satisfactory school performance and the inclusion of this individual in the environment in which they live.

One of the professionals suggested carrying out specific assessments for children under six.

"I've been trying to get the Denver test evaluated since last year. It's not a diagnostic test, it's a screening test for children under the age of six, which all children should have. So it's time for us to take the language part, remembering that it's not just speech, you have writing. [...] I'm sure we're going to have to go to a speech therapist, because it's they who treat dyscalculia, dysgraphia, retardation, dyslexia, which these kids can have like everyone else."

The literature reports that even patients with an early diagnosis of PKU and regular follow-up may present delays in neuropsychomotor development, behavioural disorders, hyperactivity, lack of attention, poor concentration, irritability, deficiencies at school and sleep problems (MONTEIRO; CÂNDIDO, 2006). The study carried out by Silva and Lamônica (2010) to assess the performance of children with PKU in the Denver-II Developmental Screening Test concluded that PKU patients diagnosed early and with good adherence to treatment performed worse in the personal-social areas, followed by the language and fine motor areas compared to non-PKU individuals.

Systematically monitoring the development of phenylketonuric children makes it possible to identify delays in good time and adopt appropriate measures. In this way, parents can realise the effects of inadequate control of blood levels of phe at an earlier stage and look for alternatives to improve this profile.

According to the professionals, the formation of operative groups is one of the strategies that has proved effective in sharing experiences and bringing everyone together, according to one of the professionals.

> "The *groups with adolescents at CEAPS, I think we have to keep doing something continuous. Going out with the adolescent on one day, just doing programming for the adolescent and reinforcing these mothers who are entering the programme. Because the mum who comes here every week needs support so she doesn't relax.*

In a study on PKU in the family, Brazier and Rowlands (2006) reported the testimony of a mother about her daughter's difficulty in ingesting the amino acid formula. She said that this moment was very stressful for the whole family and that the parents blamed themselves for thinking they had done something wrong to trigger such aversion. After observing that the problem was common to other families, they decided together to devise strategies to alleviate it. Finally, the mother reported that the group interventions had improved everyone's behaviour. The adults became less tense, and the child began to eat the protein substitute without complaints and more quickly. The mother also emphasised that it was possible to turn total refusal into acceptance.

According to Rezende et al. (2009), given the peculiarities of treatment and, in particular, adolescence, there is a need for actions aimed at adolescents, so that these young people can interact with people of the same age. The regular organisation of groups with phenylketonuric children and adults, with broad participation from the team, is also one of the service's goals. The meeting of people of the same age group, living in similar situations, can produce meaningful reflections with rich exchanges of experiences, not only strengthening the bond between them, but also enabling actions that can be implemented.

The success of treatment for individuals with chronic diseases that require specific diets is dependent on improving knowledge and changing attitudes towards the disease. However, according to Torres et aL (2009), education and the transfer of knowledge is a difficult process. As well as understanding the disease, they need to be encouraged to follow the guidelines in an ongoing educational process. In this respect, the dynamics adopted in educational groups, valuing integration and the reporting of individual experiences, can provide a strong incentive for education and adherence to treatment.

Treating patients with a late diagnosis was also considered a challenge by the professionals.

> *"There's the question of late diagnosis. Is it worth it for the family to go through all the hassle of bringing this patient here? [...] They have a chronic illness and others due to the ageing of the population. We also have to prepare for this reception, for this change in our patient's profile."*

These patients have different evolutions and impairments that are mainly related to the age at which they started treatment, the type of genetic mutation and the encouragement they receive, especially from their families.

It is known that the SUS maintains an organisational structure with an interdisciplinary logic and its challenge is to adopt Humanisation as a transversal policy, understood as a set of principles and guidelines that are translated into actions in the various health practices and spheres of the system, characterising a collective construction (BRASIL, 2011).

It's the SR's job to look for alternatives to ensure the most viable treatment in the municipalities, especially for patients with severe sequelae of the disease who find it difficult to travel to Belo Horizonte. Some of the actions demanded by families include making home visits possible, monitoring by health workers and social and psychological support for families.

Garner (2013) believes that home visits are an important mechanism for minimising the adverse effects of CD throughout childhood. Efforts in this direction should focus on increasing the capacity of carers and the community to develop healthy socio-emotional coping skills. To achieve these goals, a multidisciplinary approach of collaboration and coordination between health care, day care, early childhood education, early intervention and sectoral home visits is suggested.

Conclusions

The focus group enabled the multi-professional team to share experiences, opinions, feelings and the difficulties encountered in treating Phenylketonuria at the Reference Service.

The professionals found that most of the time families are approached abruptly when they receive the news of a change in the neonatal screening test and, after starting treatment, mothers experience feelings of anguish, denial, anger and guilt at the confirmation of a disease that will require lifelong treatment.

The team was sensitised to the disease and the treatment. Solidarity was observed between professionals, patients and family members, resulting in reciprocal affection. The bond between them increases confidence in the treatment, improves communication and favours the monitoring of phenylketonurics.

Feelings of helplessness were observed among professionals when adherence to treatment was not as expected, and integration and support among team members proved to be a strategy for sustaining the challenges presented.

The operative groups allowed the team to learn from each other and also demonstrated the importance of clarification and guidance.

The team expressed the need to decentralise treatment in order to improve the flow of care, the integration of families with health units and professionals, as well as with the community where the patients live.

Adherence to diet seems to be the crucial point in treatment, since restrictive diets can jeopardise people's lifestyles. Considering that dietary transgressions become common with advancing age, the school stage represents a major challenge for health professionals in terms of adherence to treatment. The rare and little-known disease brings difficulties in dealing with the "different" (emphasis added), which can result in conflicts and insecurity for parents.

Adolescence imposes new approaches and greater closeness to phenylketonurics on the team. This age group requires differentiated care, an even more complex experience for affected mothers and adolescents when compared to the same population without the disease.

Maternal PKU has also been a constant concern. Adolescent girls are potentially subject to this experience at an increasingly early age, requiring efforts from professionals in terms of sex education, reproduction, contraception and the prevention of sexually transmitted diseases.

The exchange of information and integration between professionals from the three sectors, the Phenylketonuria Outpatient Clinic of the SEG-HC-UFMG, the Centre for Education and Social Support (CEAPS-NUPAD) and the Treatment Control Sector (SCT) help to understand factors that interfere with treatment, as well as contributing to the improvement of the service.

This level of work requires an aggregation of knowledge, based on the perspective of comprehensive care, involving patients and their families. These factors make it possible to build collective, multidisciplinary work that points to issues that will produce knowledge about the demands presented by users and their families, in their singular and collective character.

Future research should consider the challenges of living with PKU in identifying and determining adherence to treatment in the family context. As with chronic illnesses, family interventions and interactions can act as mediators in the health process of family members.

In short, many strategies and challenges emerged during the professionals' participation in the focus group. Permanent training and integration of the team, with congruent discourses and a willingness to act, can generate productive ideas aimed at improving the treatment and quality of life of phenylketonurics and their families.

CHAPTER 8

Final considerations

"A child with phenyl is not that big of a deal,
but in quotes it is."

By giving a voice to the mothers and the professionals at the Reference Service, we realised that families' daily lives are altered by the diagnosis of Phenylketonuria (PKU) and, after this impact, parents tend to worry not only about their child's development, but also about their child's future. In this way, it was possible to understand the dimension that the disease has on the family and how it is experienced in a unique way, as a personal experience.

It is clear that PKU in the family deserves special attention, not only from a medical point of view, but also from a psychological and social perspective. It is important to recognise the feelings of helplessness, dependence and isolation that affect the family in particular.

The social isolation often present in families living with chronic illness (CD) can accentuate the vulnerability of the patient and the stigma of the disease. However, despite the suffering and difficulty of accepting the diagnosis of their child with PKU, the mothers showed positive coping attitudes and, by acquiring autonomy in relation to caring for the child, they realised that it was possible to live with the disease.

Although there are few studies on this subject, there is evidence that family relationships are fundamental to coping adequately with the disease and prolonged treatment. The need for theoretical articulation on this problem contributes to the fact that research in this area is still relatively incipient.

Meeting these unique demands requires new care practices from the team, with the family as the focus of attention to help them mobilise resources to cope and adapt. Professionals need to be attentive to identifying demands, including the family in the perspective of care, expanding spaces for dialogue and sensitive listening. Understanding this condition enables professionals to better think about their practice and recognise the complexity of care and treatment, which requires a more accurate perception of living with the disease.

The management of CD is still a challenge for professionals, and the realisation that theoretical and scientific knowledge is not enough to cover all the issues involved in treatment highlights the fragility of professional training, bringing frustration to the team.

The focus group showed that knowledge in the treatment of PKU should not be restricted to dietary prescriptions. The study points to the need to understand phenylketonurics at different stages of their development, with specific approaches according to age: infant, school, adolescent and adult. Ageing needs to be rethought, as the needs are specific to each stage of life, and CD allows for a more socialised experience, based on care.

The decentralisation of clinical/nutritional care for PKU was pointed out by professionals as a way of making treatment viable in the medium and long term, with a view to increasing the accountability of primary health care, enhancing its capacity to actively intervene. And thus gradually consolidate its legitimacy, in accordance with the institutional principles of the Unified Health System (SUS).

The study reinforces the adequacy of the concept of professional humanisation advocated by the SUS, since it contextualises this ideal in physical reality. The humanising reconstruction of health practices requires everyone to be more sensitive and attentive, open to creating bonds and taking responsibility, forming partnerships with families and mobilising possible social support networks. This work broadens this vision by including maternal perception in this precept.

It is therefore important to recognise that much remains to be done for families facing chronic conditions in childhood. We realise that the emphasis of knowledge is no longer on the concepts of health promotion and cure. The persistence of life in a state of CD weakens this ideal, while the concept of care and preservation is gaining strength in medical knowledge.

Qualitative research provides a space for political action. In this context, the methodology of this study made it possible to uncover a complex, constructed and multifaceted reality, based on the diversity found in the research subjects. It was considered that the data collection instruments were capable of revealing the reality investigated, allowing content to emerge that mirrors this population, achieving the study's objectives in a timely manner.

At the end of the study, it was possible to establish a dialogue between the two stages of the research, identifying recurring themes in the statements of the mothers interviewed and the professionals in the FG. Comparing these findings made it possible to recognise the diversity, confirming the need for professionals to deepen their knowledge, broadening their understanding of the implications of the disease on family dynamics and the aspects involved in treating phenylketonurics at different stages of life.

With the advances in knowledge about hereditary metabolic diseases, it is important to know about the need to carry out treatment that is not only focused on clinical and dietary aspects, but also on the individual experiences of patients.

Based on the results obtained, it can be concluded that Newborn Screening Programmes should also be concerned with the repercussions of the disease on the family, as well as the conditions it imposes. It should also be noted that the study's conclusions should be open to new questions, recognising the approximate nature of knowledge, a knowledge that is always unfinished.

Discussing these issues has helped to broaden our understanding of the complexity of PKU treatment and could stimulate the construction of strategies for emotional and social intervention that take into account the singularities of patients and their families. We know that ideal conditions will always be a utopia, but the search alone can lead to motivation to overcome adversity and, at the end of the journey, to rebuild and recreate a reality that will never be the same again.

The end of this work does not represent an end, but rather a new beginning, perhaps better orientated by a slightly more accurate vision, a new starting point for rethinking comprehensive care for patients with PKU.

> *"Your journey is not over yet. Reality welcomes you, telling you that the horizon of life ahead needs your words and your silence."*
>
> *(Charles Chaplin)*

CHAPTER 9

References

ACOSTA, P. B. et al. Nutrient intakes and physical growth of children with phenylketonuria undergoing nutrition therapy. *J Am Diet Assoe,* Chicago, v. 103, n. 9, p. 1167-1173, Sept. 2003.

ACOSTA, P. B.; YANNICELLI, S. *The Ross metabolic formula system, nutrition support protocols.* 4th ed. Columbus: Ross Laboratories, 2001.

AGUIAR, M. J. B. Genetic Services and research in the State of Minas Gerais, Brazil. *Comm genet,* Basel, v. 7, n. 2-3, p. 117-120, Nov. 2004.

ALAEI, M. et al. Family Social Status and Dietary Adherence of Patients with Phenylketonuria. *Iran J Pediatr,* Tehran, v. 21, n. 3, p. 379-384, Sept. 2011.

ALVES-MAZZOTTI, A. J.; GEWANDSZNAJDER, F. O *Método nas ciências naturais e sociais:* pesquisa quantitativa e qualitativa. 2 ed.

ARAÚJO, C. A.; MELLO, M. A.; RIOS, A. M. G. *Resilience:* theory and research practices in psychology. São Paulo: Ithaka Books, 2011.

ARAÚJO, H. M. C.; ARAÚJO, W. M. C.; BOTELHO, R. B. A.; ZANDONADI, R. P. Celiac disease, eating habits and practices and quality of life. *RevNutr,* Campinas, v. 23, n. 3, p. 467-474, May/June, 2010.

ARAÚJO, Y. B. et al. Fragility of the social network of families of children with chronic illness. *Rev Bras Enferm,* Brasília, v. 66, n. 5, p. 675-81, Sep/Oct 2013.

ARCHER, L. A.; CUNNINGHAM, C. E, WHELAN, D. T. Coping with dietary in Phenylketonuria: a case report. *Canadian Journal of Behavioral Science,* Saskatoon, v. 20, n.4, p. 461-466, Oct. 1988.

AWISZUS, D.; UNGER, I. Coping with PKU: results of narrative interviews with parents. *Eur J Pediatr,* Berlin, v. 149, n. 1, p. 45-51, Jan. 1990.

BARDIN, L. *Content analysis.* Lisbon: Edições 70, 2011,223p.

BEKHOF, J. et al. Influence of knowledge of the disease on metabolic contracti in phenylketonuria. *EurJ Pediatr,* Berlin, v. 162, n. 6, p. 440- 442, june 2003.

BERGMAN, A.S.; LEWISTON, N.J.; WEST, A.M. Social work practice and chronic paediatric illness. *Soc Work Health Care,* New York, v. 4, n. 3, p. 265-274, Spring 1979.

BONN, M. J. L. Phenylketonuria. Switzerland: Annales Nestlé, 2010. 88 p.

BOOG M. C. F. Nutritional education: past, present and future. *Rev Nutr,* Campinas, v. 10, n. 1, p. 5-19, jan./jun. 1997.

BOOG, M. C. F. Qualitative research in the field of food and nutrition. In: BARROS, N. F.; CECATTI, J. G.; TURATO, E. R. (Org.). Qualitative research in health: multiple perspectives. Campinas: Komedi, 2005. p. 97-108.

BOOG, M. C. F. Atuação do nutricionista em saúde pública na promoção da alimentação saudável. *Revista Ciência e Saúde*, Porto Alegre, v. 1, n.1, p 33-42, jan./jun. 2008.

BOOG, M. C. F. Nutritional education in public health services. *Cad Saúde Pública*, Rio e Janeiro, v. 15, (supl. 2), p. 139-147, 1999.

BRAZIL. Federal Law 8069 of 13 July 1990. Provides for the Statute of the Child and Adolescent. *Federal Official Gazette*, Brasília, 16 July 1990. Available at: <www.presidencia.gov.br/CCivil/Leis/L8069.htm>. Accessed on: 25 January 2010.

BRAZIL. Ministry of Health. National Health Surveillance Agency. *Clarifications on Phenylketonuria* (Technical Report No. 49, 11 April 2012). Available at: <http://portal.anvisa.gov.br>. Accessed on: 25 November 2013.

BRAZIL. Ministry of Health, Secretariat of Health Care, Department of Specialised Care. Manual of technical standards and operational routines of the National Neonatal Screening Programme Brazil. 2. ed. Brasília: Ministério da Saúde; 2005.

BRAZIL. Ministry of Health. Health Care Secretariat. *National Policy for the Humanisation of SUS Health Care and Work Management.* Brasília: Ministry of Health, 2011. Series F. Communication and Health Education.

BRAZIL. Ministry of Health. Health Care Secretariat. *National Policy for the Humanisation of SUS Health Care and Work Management.* Extended and Shared Clinic Brasília: Ministry of Health, 2009. Series B. Basic Health Texts.

BRAZIER, A.; ROWLANDS, C. PKU in the family: working together. *Clin Child Psychol Psychiatry*, London, v. 11, n. 3, p. 483-488, July 2006.

BURGARD, P. Family conditions and dietary control in IEMs. *J Inherit Metab Dis*, Dordrecht, v. 30, n. 5, p. 629, Oct. 2007.

CANGUILHEM, G. The *Normal and the Pathological.* 6. ed. São Paulo: Editora Forense Universitária, 2006, 293p.

CAREGNATO, R. C. A.; MUTTI, R. Qualitative research: discourse analysis versus content analysis . *Texto contexto-enferm*, Florianópolis, v. 15, n. 4, p. 679-684, Oct./Dec. 2006.

CARVAJAL, G. *Becoming an adolescent:* the adventure of a metamorphosis. São Paulo: Cortez, 2001.

CARVALHO, C. S. U. A necessária atenção à família do paciente oncológico. *Revista Brasileira de Cancerologia*, Rio de Janeiro, v. 54, n. 1, p. 87-96, 2008.

CASTRO, E. K.; PICCININI, C. A. Implications of chronic organic disease in childhood for family relationships: some theoretical issues. *Psicologia: Reflexão e Crítica*, Porto Alegre, v. 15, n. 3, p. 625-635, 2002.

CASTRO, I. P. S. et al. Relationships between phenylalanine leveis, Intelligence and socioeconomic status of patients with phenylketonuria. *Jornal de Pediatria*, Rio de Janeiro, v. 88, n. 4, p. 353-356, 2012.

CECÍLIO, L. C. O. et al. Primary health care and the construction of thematic health networks: what role can it play? *Ciência e Saúde Coletiva.* Rio de Janeiro, v. 17, n. 11, 2893-2902, 2012.

CLARK, B. J. After a positive Guthrie - what next? Dietary management for the child with phenylketonuria. *Eur J ClinNutr,* Basingstoke, v. 46, p. 33-39, june 1992.

CLAVREUL, J. *A ordem médica:* poder e impotência do discurso médico. Editora Brasiliense: São Paulo, 1983. 275p.

CORNEJO, V.; RAIMANN, E. Inborn errors of amino acid metabolism. In: COLOMBO, M.; CORNEJO, V.; RAIMANN, E. *Errores Innatos en el Metabolismo Del Nino.* 3. ed. Santiago de Chile: Universitaria, 2010. p. 65- 75.

CRONE, M. R. et al. Behavioural factors related to metabolic control in patients with phenylketonuria. *J Inherit Metab Dis,* Dordrecht, v. 28, n. 5, 627-37, 2005.

DAMIÃO, E.; ÂNGELO, M. The family's experience of living with a child's chronic illness. *Rev Esc EnfUSP,* São Paulo, v. 35, n. 1, p. 66-71,2001.

DEMO, P. Pesquisa qualitativa: busca de equilíbrio entre forma e conteúdo. *Rev Latino-Am Enfermagem,* Ribeirão Preto, v. 6, n. 2, p. 89-104, April 1998.

DENZIM, N. K. *The research act in sociology:* a theoretical introduction to sociological methods. London: Butterworth, 1970.

DI CIOMMO, V.; FORCELLA, E.; COTUGO, G. Living with phenylketonuria from the point of view of children, adolescents, and young adults: a qualitative study. *J Dev Behav Pediatr,* Baltimore, v. 33, n. 3, p. 229-235, April 2012.

FERREIRA, H. P. et al. The impact of chronic illness on the carer. *Revista Brasileira Clínica Médica,* São Paulo, v. 10, n. 4, p. 278-284, 2012.

FERREIRA, R. A. et al. Adolescents: particularities of care. In: LEÃO, E. et al. *Outpatient Paediatrics.* 5. ed. Belo Horizonte: Coopmed, 2013. p. 153-169.

FIESE, B. H.; EVERHART, R. S. Medication adherence and childhood chronic illness: family daily management skills and emotional climate as emerging contributors. *CurrOpin Pediatr,* Philadelphia, v. 18, n. 5, p. 551-557, 2006.

FONTANELLA, B. J. B.; CAMPOS, C. J. G.; TURATO, E. R. Data collection in clinical-qualitative research: use of non-directed interviews with open questions by health professionals. *Rev Latino-Am Enfermagem,* Ribeirão Preto, v. 14, n. 5, 2006.

FONTANELLA, B. J. B; RICAS, J, TURATO, E. R. Saturation sampling in qualitative health research: theoretical contributions. *Cad. Saúde Pública,* Rio de Janeiro, v. 24, n. 1, p. 17-27, 2008.

FRANK, N.; FITZGERALD, R.; LEGGE, M. Phenylketonuria: the lived experience. *N ZMed J,* Wellington, NewZealand, v. 120, n. 1262, Sept. 2007.

FREIRE, P. *Pedagogia da autonomia:* saberes necessárias à prática educativa. 28. ed., São Paulo: Editora Paz e Terra, 2003, 148p.

GARCIA, R. W. D.; CANESQUI, A. M. (Org.) *Anthropology and Nutrition:* a possible dialogue. Rio de Janeiro: Editora FIOCRUZ, 2005 (Anthropology and Health Collection).

GARNER, A. S. Home visiting and the biology of toxic stress: opportunities to address early childhood adversity. *Pediatrics,* Elk Grove Village, v. 132, Suppl 2, p. S65-73, 2013.

GOFFMAN, E. Stigma: notes on deteriorated manipulation. 4. ed. Rio de Janeiro: LTC S.S., 1988, 124p.

GOMES, R. Data analysis in qualitative research. In: MINAYO M. D. S. (Org.). *Pesquisa social:* teoria, método e criatividade. Petrópolis: Vozes, 1999. p. 67-80.

GREVE, L. C. et al. *Breast-feeding in the management of the newborn with phenylketonuria:* a practical approach to dietary therapy. *J Am Diet* Assoe, Sacramento, v. 94, p. 305-309, mar. 1994.

GUTIERREZ, D. M. D.; MINAYO, M. C. S. Production of knowledge on health care within the family. *Ciência e Saúde Coletiva.* Rio de Janeiro, v. 15, n. 1, p. 1497-1508, 2010.

HOROVITZ, D. D. G.; LLERENA JR., J. C.; MATTOS, R. A. Attention to birth defects in Brazil: current panorama. *Cad. Saúde Pública,* Rio de Janeiro, v. 21, n. 4, p. 1055-1064, 2005.

HUIJBREGTS, S. C. J. et al. Short-term dietary interventions in children and adolescents with treated phenylketonuria: effects on neuropsychological outcome of a well-controlled population. *J Inherit Metab Dis,* Dordrecht, v. 25, n. 6, p. 419- 430, Oct. 2002.

IERVOLINO, S. A.; PELICIONI, M. C. F. The use of focus groups as a qualitative methodology in health promotion. *Rev Esc Enf,* São Paulo, v. 35, n. 2, p. 115-21,2001.

JANUÁRIO, J. N. Neonatal screening. In: LEÃO, E. et al. *Outpatient Paediatrics.* 5. ed. Belo Horizonte: Coopmed, 2013. p. 117-122.

KANUFRE, V. C. et al. Dietary Approach to Phenylketonuria. *Revista Médica de Minas Gerais,* Belo Horizonte, v. 11, n. 3, p. 129-134, 2001a.

KANUFRE, V. C. et al. Phenylketonuria and the special diet: a challenge for maintaining body weight. *Revista Médica de Minas Gerais,* Belo Horizonte, v. 20, n. 4, p. 20-24, 2010. Supplement 3.

KANUFRE, V. C.; SANTOS, J. S.; SOARES, R. D. L.; REIS, D. G. *Special recipes for Phenylketonuria.* Belo Horizonte: Folium, 2001b.

KITZINGER, J. Focus groups with users and health care professionals. In: POPE, C.; MAYS, N. *Pesquisa qualitativa na atenção à saúde.* 2. ed. Porto Alegre: Artmed, 2006. p. 31-40.

KÚBLER-ROSS, E. *Sobre a morte e o morrer.* 8 ed. São Paulo: Martins Fontes, 2000, 299p.

MACDONALD, A. et al. The reality of dietary compliance in the management of phenylketonuria. *J Inherit Metab Dis,* Dordrecht, v. 33, n. 6, p. 665-670, dec. 2010.

MARTINS, A. M. et al. *Brazilian Dietary Protocol:* inborn errors of metabolism. São Paulo: Segmento Farma editores, 2006.

MARTINS, A. M.; FISBERG, M. R. V.; SCHIMIDT B. J. *Fenilcetonúria:* abordagem terapêutica. São Paulo: Nestlé, 1993. (Nestlé Paediatrics Topics).

MARTINS, S. R. R. *Incidence of Phenylketonuria and other hyperphenylalaninemias in the State of Minas Gerais:* data from the State Neonatal Screening Programme. 2005. 98 f. Dissertation (Master's in Child and Adolescent Health Sciences) - School of Medicine, Universidade Federal de Minas Gerais, Belo Horizonte, 2005.

MINAYO, M. C. S. Qualitative analysis: theory, steps and reliability. *Ciênc saúde coletiva,* Rio de Janeiro, v. 17, n. 3, p. 621-626, mar. 2012.

MINAYO, M. C. de S. O *desafio do conhecimento:* Pesquisa qualitativa em saúde. 8. ed. São Paulo: Hucitec, 2004, 269p.

MINAYO, M. C. S. et al. *Pesquisa social:* teoria, método e criatividade. 24. ed. Petrópolis: Vozes, 1994, 80p.

MIRA, N. V. M.; MARQUEZ, U. M. L. Importância do diagnóstico e tratamento da Fenilcetonúria. *Rev. Saúde Pública,* São Paulo, v. 34, n. 1, p. 86-96, 2000.

MONTEIRO, L. T. B.; CÂNDIDO, L. M. B. Phenylketonuria in Brazil: evolution and cases. *Rev Nutr,* Campinas, v. 19, n. 3, p. 381-387, May/Jun. 2006.

MOREIRA, P. L.; DUPAS, G. Living with diabetes: the experience told by the child. *Rev. Latino-Am. Enfermagem,* Ribeirão Preto, v. 14, n. 1, p. 25-32, jan./feb. 2006.

MORGAN, D. L. *Focus Groups as Qualitative Research.* 2nd ed. Thousand Oaks, CA, US: Sage Publications, 1997. (Qualitative Research Methods, v. 16)

NALIN, T. et al. Phenylketonuria in the Unified Health System: evaluation of adherence to treatment in a care centre in Rio Grande do Sul. *Rev. HCPA,* Porto Alegre, v. 30, n. 3, p. 225-232, 2010.

NATIONAL INSTITUTES OF HEALTH CONSENSUS DEVELOPMENT PANEL. Phenylketonuria: screening and management. *Pediatrics,* Elk Grove Village, v. 108, n. 4, p. 972-982, oct. 2001.

NAZARETH, C. A. L.; SOUZA, L. A.; FIGUEIREDO, M. A. G. *Art as a strategy for health education:* a waiting room experience. Juiz de Fora: Editar, 2007.

NEVES, J. L. Pesquisa qualitativa: pesquisa, usos e possibilidades. *Caderno de pesquisas em administração,* São Paulo, v. 1, n. 3, p. 1-5, 1993.

NÓBREGA, V. M. et al. Impositions and conflicts in the daily lives of families of children with chronic illness. *EscAnna Nery,* Rio de Janeiro, v. 14, n. 4, p. 781- 788, Oct./Dec. 2012.

PAPALIA, D. E.; OLDS, S. W. *Desenvolvimento Humano. 7.* ed. Porto Alegre: Artes Médicas Sul, 2000.

PERRICONE, G. et al. Functioning of family system in paediatric oncology during treatment phase. *Paediatr Hematol Oncol,* London, V. 29, n. 7, p. 652-662, 2012.

PERRICONE, G. et al. Maternal coping strategies in response to a child's chronic and oncological disease: a cross-cultural study in Italy and Portugal. *Pediatric Reports,* Palermo, v. 5, e11, p. 43-47, 2013.

PIETZ, J. et al. No Evidence for Individual Blood-Brain Barrier Phenylketonuria Transport to Influence Clinicai Outcome in Typical Phenylketonuria Patients. *Ann Neurol,* Boston, v. 52, n. 3, p. 120-128, Sept. 2002.

PIRES, A. P. *Communicating bad news.* Porto Alegre, 1998. Available at: <www.ufrgs.br/bioetica/masnot.htm>. Accessed on: 28 February 2014.

POPE, C.; MAYS, N. *Pesquisa qualitativa na atenção à saúde. 2.* ed. Porto Alegre: Artmed, 2006, 118p.

REZENDE, A. M.; SCHALL, V. T.; MODENA, C. M. Adolescence and becoming ill: the experience of an adolescent with cancer. *Aletheia,* Canoas, v. 30, p. 88-100, 2009.

RIGOTTO, R. M. The techniques of oral reports and the study of social representations in health. *Ciênc Saúde Coletiva,* Rio de Janeiro, v. 3, n. 1, p. 116-129, 1998.

RODRIGUES, E. M.; BOOG, M. C. F. Affective experience with food: sensitisation strategy in educational action with obese adolescents. *Nutrição em Pauta, v. 72,* p. 41-45, May/June, 2005.

ROMANELLI, G. The meaning of food in the family: an anthropological view. *Medicina,* Ribeirão Preto, v. 39, n. 3, p. 333-339, jul./set. 2006.

RUSSEL, F. F" MILLS, B. C" ZUCCONI, T. Relationship of parental attitudes and knowledge to treatment adherence in children with PKU. *Pediatr Nurs,* Pitman NJ, v. 14, n. 6, p. 514-516, 523, 1988.

SANTOS, S. V. *A família da criança com doença chónica:* Abordagem de algumas características. *Análise Psicológica,* Lisbon, v. 1, n. 16, p. 65-75, 1998.

SCHILD, S. Parents of children with PKU. *Child Today,* Washington, v. 1, n. 4, p. 20-22, 1972.

SCHWEITZER-KRANTZ S" BURGARD P. Survey of national guidelines for the treatment of phenylketonuria. *Eur J Pediatr,* Berlin, v. 159, Suppl 2, p. 70-73, 2000.

SCRIVER, C. R.; KAUFMAN, S. Hyperphenylalaninaemia: phenylalanine hydroxylase deficiency. In: SCRIVER, C. R. et al. *The metabolic and molecular basis of inherited disease.* 8. ed. New York: McGraw-Hill, 2001. p. 1667-1724.

SHAW, V.; LAWSON, M. Disorders of amino acid metabolism, organic acidaemias and urea cycles defects. In: . *Clinicai paediatric dietetics.* London: Blackwell Science, 1994, p. 177-209.

SILVA, F. M.; CORRÊA, I. Chronic Illness in Childhood: the Family Member's Experience of the Child's Hospitalisation. *Revista Mineira de Enfermagem,* Belo Horizonte, v. 10, n. 1, p. 18-23, 2006.

SILVA, G. K.; LAMÔNICA, D. A. C. Performance of children with Phenylketonuria in the Denver Developmental Screening Test - II. *Pró-Fono R Atual Cient,* São Paulo, v. 22, n. 1, p. 345-50, 2010.

SILVA, M. A. S. et al. Family daily life in coping with chronic conditions in childhood. *Acta Paul Enferm,* São Paulo, v. 23, n. 3, p. 359-65, 2010.

SIMIONI, A. M. C.; LEFÈVRE, F.; PEREIRA, I. M. T. B. *Metodologia qualitativa nas pesquisas em saúde coletiva:* considerações teóricas e instrumentais. São Paulo: USP, 1996. 15p.

SIMON, E. et al. Evaluation of quality of life and description of sociodemographic state in adolescent and young adult patients with phenylketonuria. *Health Qual Life Outcomes,* London, v. 6, n. 25, p. 1-7, 2008.

SMITH, I.; LEE, P. The Hyperphenylalaninaemias. In: FERNANDES, J. *et al.* (Ed.). *Inborn metabolic diseases diagnosis and treatment.* 3. ed. Berlin: Springer, p. 171- 184, 2000.

SMITH, I.; BEASLEY, I. M. G.; ADES, A. E. Intelligence and quality of dietary treatment in phenylketonuria. *Archives of Disease in Childhood,* London, v. 65, p. 472-478, 1990.

SOARES, S. M.; FERRAZ, A. F. Operative learning groups in health services: Systematisation of foundations and methodologies. *Esc Anna Nery R Enferm,* Rio de Janeiro, v. 11, n. 1, p. 52-57, 2007.

STARLING, A. L. P. *et al. Understanding Phenylketonuria:* Guidance Manual. Belo Horizonte: Editora UFMG, 2006. 37p.

STARLING, A. L. P. Phenylketonuria: diagnosis and treatment. *Revista Médica de Minas Gerais,* Belo Horizonte, v. 15, n. 3, p. 187-189, 2005.

STARLING, A. L. P.; AGUIAR, M. J. B.; KANUFRE, V. C. Phenylketonuria. *Revista Médica de Minas Gerais,* Belo Horizonte, v. 9, n. 3, p. 106-110, 1999.

SULLIVAN, J. E.; CHANG, P. Review: Emotional and behavioural functioning in Phenylketonuria. *J Pediatr Psychol,* Cary NC, v. 24, n. 3, p. 281-299, 1999.

SURTEES, R.; BLAU, N. The neurochemistry of phenylketonuria. *Eur J Pediatr,* Berlin, v. 159, n. 2, p. 109-113, Oct. 2000.

TOMAZI, N. G. S.; YAMAMOTO, R. M. *Metodologia de pesquisa em saúde:* fundamentos essenciais. Curitiba: Autores Paranaenses, 1999. 98 p.

TORAL, N.; SLATER, B. Transtheoretical model approach to eating behaviour. *Ciênc. saúde coletiva,* v. 12, n. 6, p. 1641-1650, nov./dez, 2007.

TORRES, H. C. et al. Strategic evaluation of group and individual education in the diabetes education programme. *Rev. Saúde Pública,* São Paulo, v. 43, n. 2, p. 291-298, 2009.

TRIVINOS, A. N. S. *Introdução à pesquisa em ciências sociais:* a pesquisa qualitativa em educação. São Paulo: Atlas, 1994. 175p.

TURATO, E. R. *Tratado de metodologia da pesquisa clínico qualitativa:* construção teórico epistemológica, discussão comparada e aplicação nas áreas de saúde e humanas. 2. ed. Petrópolis: Vozes, 2003.

TURATO, E. R.; FONTANELLA, B. J. B.; CAMPOS, C. J. G. *Data collection in clinical-qualitative research:* use of non-directed interviews with open questions by health professionals. *Rev. Latino-Am Enfermagem,* v. 14, n. 5, 2006.

VIEIRA, M. A.; LIMA, R. A. G. Children and adolescents with chronic illness: Living with changes. *Rev. Latino-Am. Enfermagem,* Ribeirão Preto, v. 10, n. 4, p. 552-560, 2002.

WAISBREN, S. E. et al. Social factors and the meaning of food in adherence to medicated diets: results of a maternal phenylketonuria summercamp. *J Inher Metab Dis,* Dordrecht, v. 20, n. 1, p. 21-27, jan. 1997.

WALDOW, V. R.; BORGES, R. F. Caring and humanising: relationships and meanings. *Acta Paul Enferm,* São Paulo, v. 24, n.3, p. 414-418, 2011.

WAPPNER, R. et al. Management of phenylketonuria for optimal outcome: a review of guidelines for phenylketonuria management and report of surveys of parents, patients, and clinic directors. *Pediatrics,* Elk Grove Village, v. 104, n. 6, Dec. 1999.

WEGLAGE, J. et al. Behavioural and emotional problems in early-treat adolescents with Phenylketonuria in comparison with diabetic patients and health contrais. *J Inherit Metab Dis,* Dordrecht, v. 23, n. 5, p. 487-496, 2000.

WEGLAGE, J; RUPP, A.; SCHMIDT, E. Personality characteristics in patients with phenylketonuria treated erly. *Pediatric Research,* Baltimore. v. 35, n. 5, p. 611-613, 1994.

WORLD HEALTH ORGANISATION (WHO). *Adherence to long-term therapies:* evidence for action. Geneva: World Health Organisation, 2003. Available at: <http://www.who.int/chp/knowledge/publications/adherence_report/en/index.htm   I>. Accessed on: 18 June 2007.

YUNES, M. A. M. *Positive psychology and resilience:* the focus on the individual and the family. *Psicologia em estudo,* Maringá, v. 8, p. 75-84, 2003. Special issue.

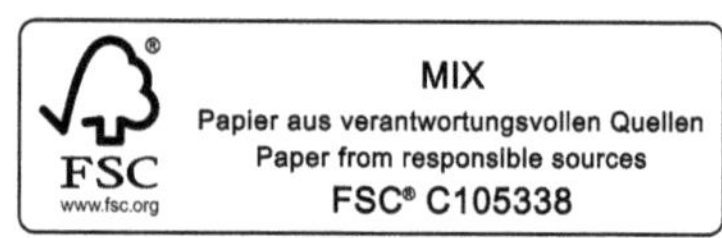

Printed by Books on Demand GmbH, Norderstedt / Germany